Colby Arie Hadily Nerissa Shane
Forgiveness Baby Mercy Bowen Wes
Nadia Gabriel Pearl Crystal Elizabeth
Christian Cheyenne Davis William
Jacob Noel Austin Genia Jonathan
Larsen Baby Johnson Baby Luczek
ich Baby Hays Laura Danny Sarah
ancock Baby Homan Baby Baumli
k Baby Berens Baby Leinart Pete
y Charles Baby Stevens Baby Wood
zales Baby Verbrugge Vincent Ellorie
x Baby Darr Baby Besher Daniel

Samuel Sable Maddie Maxie Bab

Seth Jericho Sam James Peter Baby

Alyssa Kiara Gracie Lily Ember Hol

Morgan Laura Linda Rachel Krist

Kelsey Joshua Tina Scott Jodi Garr

Molly Baby Young Baby Miller B

Baby Perry Reed Daniel Baby Sank

Baby Emmorey Baby Gritter Baby

Baby Kent Baby Bullock Baby F

Austin Rebekah Gregory Baby Moc

Lisa Evan Holly Gary Katelyn Baby

Baby Nichols Baby Carpenter Baby

To:

_____

From:

_____

Date:

_____

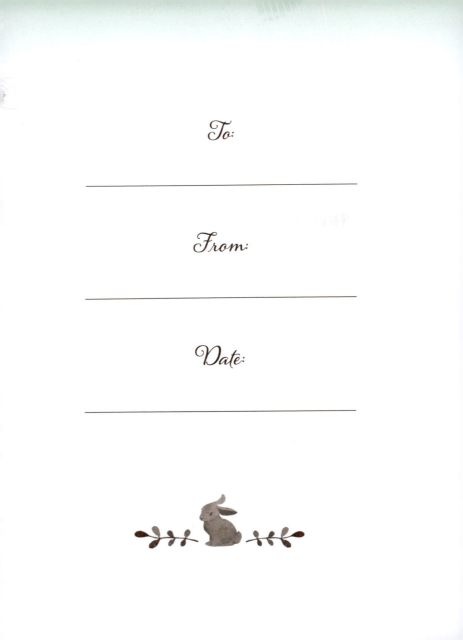

"One of the most confounding and lonely events in our lives is the death of an unborn child. It seems as if such a loss doesn't 'count' as so many around us either don't understand or don't even know of our grief. But the grief is real. And life-changing. Kathe provides a tender and helpful book to offer companionship, help, and hope in such a time."

—Elisa Morgan, speaker, author of *The Beauty of Broken* and *Hello, Beauty Full*, and co-host of *Discover the Word*

"*Grieving the Child I Never Knew* was the only book I connected with after the loss of my twins. Kathe Wunnenberg was one of my inspirations for starting Owl Love You Forever, a nonprofit providing boxes to hospitals for families who lose a baby. I include a copy of this devotional in each of our boxes. There's something incredibly powerful about having the text in your hands when you need it and room to journal as you heal."

—Shayla Van Hofwegen, founder and president of Owl Love You Forever

"I am so thankful that God has used Kathe to write this devotional for parents who have lost a child. This devotional walks a grieving parent through the journey of grief in such a comforting way. *Grieving the Child I Never Knew* helps a grieving parent heal from the inside out. I would recommend this book to anyone who has lost a child. They will be blessed beyond measure."

—Heather Gillis, author of *Waiting for Heaven* and founder of Bowen's Hope Foundation

"*Grieving the Child I Never Knew* is a book that's been needed for a long time. I've always referred to it as the silent journey. People are uncomfortable talking about it. They make trite comments as though that will help you through your grief. I have watched my daughter lose three babies, all at different stages. Her grief has been palatable. I appreciate the format of this book. A devotional book, designed for the reader to use however it best fits her present need. I highly recommend this book not only for women who have had to walk this journey of grief, but for all women to better understand those who do."

—Donna Fagerstrom, women's ministry leader of Converge Worldwide

GRIEVING
THE
Child
I NEVER KNEW

A Devotional for Comfort
in the Loss of Your Unborn or Newly Born Child

KATHE WUNNENBERG

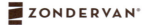 ZONDERVAN®

Grieving the Child I Never Knew

© 2001, 2015 by Kathe Wunnenberg

Requests for information should be addressed to:

Zondervan, *3900 Sparks Dr. SE, Grand Rapids, MI 49546*

ISBN 978-0-310-35065-1

Printed in China

16 17 18 19 TIMS 6 5 4 3 2

*To my children I never knew but
who have left an eternal imprint in my life:
Zachary, John Samuel, Luke, and Matthew*

And to yours . . .

✦ Contents ✦

Eight Ways to Use This Book   xi

Readings for Special Days or Needs   xv

Introduction   xvii

Part 1: Hiding

   1. Hide-and-Seek   2

   2. Journey to the Hiding Place   6

   3. Facing the Truth   11

   4. From Minimizing to Validating   18

   5. Missing in Action   23

Part 2: Suffering

   6. Nothing to Show for My Loss   30

   7. Journey Through the Darkness
      of Depression   35

   8. The Empty Frame   40

9. Happy-Sad Days   46

10. Husbands and Wives Grieve Differently   51

PART 3: QUESTIONING

11. Drowning in the Sea of Why   60

12. Why Am I So Angry?   65

13. Why Do I Feel So Guilty?   72

14. God, Where Are You?   77

15. Jesus Has a Rocking Chair   83

PART 4: FORGIVING

16. Hidden Unforgiveness   90

17. Forgiving Others   95

18. Journey to the Snowdrift
    of Forgiving Yourself   103

19. Forgiving God   109

20. Receiving the Gift of Forgiveness   116

PART 5: RELATING

21. Who Do You Say That I Am?   126

22. He'll Meet You Where You Are   131

23. Journey Through the Seasons
    of Friendship   137

24. Playmates in Heaven   144

25. It's Pitcher-Filling Time!   149

PART 6: SEEKING
    26. Seeing Beyond Your Cloud of Loss   158
    27. Do You Want to Get Well?   164
    28. Holding Hands with Your Future   170
    29. Journey Through the Gallery of Praise   178
    30. Seeking Others Before You, Beside You,
        Behind You   183
    31. I'll Know My Child in Heaven   189

PART 7: SHARING YOUR STORY   195

A Prayer Guide for Special Days   199

Discussion Guide   208

Scripture Index   214

A Note from the Author   216

⚜ Eight Ways to ⚜
Use This Book

*G*rieving the Child I Never Knew is not a how-to book with pat answers about grieving the loss of a child. My hope is that this book will become your personal companion. Think of it as a trusted friend who walks beside you and gives you permission to be who you are and where you are in your journey. If you are hiding your pain or hiding from people, then discover how God will meet you in your isolation. If you are suffering and need to cry, then weep with all your heart. If you feel like relating to others to help them through a similar journey, then connect. And if you are seeking hope, help, and healing to press on in your future, then start today.

Whether you've recently suffered loss or lost a child long ago, my prayer is that *Grieving the Child I Never Knew* will be a tool to guide you to a deeper understanding of who God is and will meet you in the pain of your loss and point you to Him.

Grieving the Child I Never Knew contains thirty-one devotions divided into six parts. Each devotion contains a scripture passage, a practical or biblical illustration, a prayer, discussion questions, and space for journaling. Part 7 includes a guide for sharing your story. Additional resources are listed at the back of the book to encourage you in your healing journey.

How you choose to use this book depends on your unique personality, needs, and desired outcomes. Consider the following possible "settings," and choose the one that feels most comfortable to you.

Your 31-Day Companion. This devotional can be your personal companion for the next month. Whether you choose to curl up with your book in bed each night, start your day with it at the breakfast table, or take a break with it at work, you decide the time and place that's best for you.

Quick Pick-Me-Up. Keep your devotional on the coffee table, ready and available for you to pick up when questions or emotions surface and you need a quick dose of encouragement. Use the table of contents as a compass to guide you to the reading that meets your needs in the moment.

Table for Two. Heartfelt conversation with another person can double your insights, laughter, and tears. Sitting with someone can give you courage and motivation to finish the book. Who will join you at the table? Your spouse? Friend? Neighbor? Coworker? Family member? Pastor? Counselor? The person you know who lost a child too?

Grief Group Discussion Guide. Your devotional can be a tool to facilitate grief discussions in small or large groups. The options are endless. Choose the format, readings, and number of weeks that meet your group's needs, or use the discussion guide at the end of this book.

Small-Group Bible Study. Use the devotional as a six-week Bible study for anyone who desires to know more about grieving the loss of a child. Focus on one section per week. Have your group memorize Scripture from the readings.

A Gift That Lasts. Someone you know has lost a child. Make this devotional your treasured gift for the bereaved. Share how this book has encouraged you in your journey.

A Resource Book for Pastors and Counselors. When someone dies, pastors and counselors are usually the first people called. This devotional guide can accompany them as they meet with the bereaved and can be given as a gift that says they care.

A Prayer Guide. Praying God's Word is a powerful gift you can give or receive. This addition at the back of the book will guide prayers on special days and occasions. Pray for yourself, pray for others, or enlist others to pray God's Word for you. The next time someone asks, "How can I encourage you?" invite him or her to use the prayer guide in this book and pray for you!

Readings for
Special Days or Needs

Special occasions, holidays, and personal circumstances may trigger your grief and expose a new dimension of grieving your child. When you encounter these times in your journey and desire encouragement or a fresh perspective, turn to the selected reading for that specific day or need.

Mother's Day 11, 46, 83, 126, 178

Father's Day. 46, 83, 170

Grandparents Day 46

Anniversary/Birthday 46, 131, 189

Due date 46

Helping children grieve 46, 60, 131, 198

Helping couples cope 18, 51, 65, 72, 83, 170, 189

Grandparents who grieve 40, 46, 72, 126, 189

Holidays/family gatherings . . . 11, 40, 46, 65, 116, 126

Trying to have another child . . . . xvii, 158, 164

INTRODUCTION

I never knew this child fully, so why do I grieve so deeply? I never held this tiny baby, never saw the sleeping face, never locked eyes and gazed into the soul of this little person. Yet I feel as if a part of me died and left a void in my being. Most people don't seem to understand and minimize my loss instead of validating my pain from losing this nameless child. Will I always feel so lonely and misunderstood? Is it normal to mourn someone I never knew or lost so long ago? How can I move beyond the hurt and begin to hope again? Only when I gave myself permission to grieve the loss of my child did I begin to pick up the pieces of my broken heart and start to heal.

My journey through grieving the child I never knew began when I stepped back through my memories to a time early in my marriage when my husband and I decided to start a family. I expected to have a child within a year, just like everyone else I knew. To my surprise, I discovered that conceiving a child didn't come easily for me. Two years, numerous doctor visits, months of temperature charts, and many ovulation kits later, I finally discovered I was pregnant just days before Christmas. I didn't realize at the time that God would use this unknown child to penetrate my heart and draw me close to Him in a way I had never experienced.

When I lost our baby on my husband's thirtieth birthday, I was disappointed but didn't feel deeply about this loss. Why should I? I never knew this child. Unaware that my pain was hidden and my journey through grief had already begun, I pressed on in life.

About two years later, God fulfilled the desires of our heart by providing us a baby through a Christian adoption agency. When our son Jake was a toddler, he began to pray for "a baby to grow in Mommy's belly." I was shocked. But he persisted. A couple of years later, when I went to the doctor for the "flu," he announced, "You're pregnant!" Jake knew that God had answered his prayer.

But a few weeks later, on Good Friday, our family stared at the monitor in disbelief, realizing our unborn baby had a fatal birth defect. I found myself in my own Garden of Gethsemane, crying out, "God, please take this cup of suffering from me!" By Easter morning, I released my anguish and my unborn child into His care. "Not my will, but Yours be done!"

During the long months of waiting on the birth of my baby, God worked through this child to teach me many life lessons. On different days I laughed, cried, learned the necessity of silence and solitude, released control, allowed others to encourage me, and saw my faith soar. I tasted humility and surrender, and I learned what it means to enjoy every moment. I learned how precious praying friends are, and I learned how faithful and loving God is to care about me personally.

I didn't know what the future held, but I was certain of *who* held the future. I believed God was able to heal my child—and I proclaimed that publicly. Yet I also knew that if He chose not to, I would praise Him anyway! On August 22, our son John Samuel was born with eyes looking up at God. His birth was a celebration of God's love and a testimony of the value of every life. Within a few hours, heaven's gates opened and welcomed him into the arms of Jesus. His brief life touched thousands of people with the reality of God, and the ripple effects will be known only in eternity.

A few months later, I discovered I was pregnant again. *How caring of God to bless me with another child!* I thought. But I never got to know this child or hold this baby in my arms. A few weeks into my pregnancy, I miscarried. My heart was breaking for all three children I had lost.

Then a few months later, I discovered I was pregnant again! *Surely God will allow me to keep this child!* I thought. But He didn't. On Christmas Eve I lost this child too. "Where are You, God?" I cried out. God used this fourth child I lost to help me grieve openly and share my pain with others through writing about grief.

When the doctor confirmed that I was pregnant with a fifth child, I was terrified at the thought of another loss. But God overshadowed my fear with faith to trust Him yet another time. Joshua was born healthy—after nearly nineteen years of marriage. Two years later, another son, Jordan, was born when I was forty-two. Although my journey is different from yours and I may never fully understand everything you are feeling, I can relate to some of your pain. Behind the pages of this book is an ordinary woman and a fellow griever, still in the journey of grieving the loss of four children. And behind the woman is a faithful God who has made this book possible. My prayer is that *Grieving the Child I Never Knew* will help point you to God and that you will experience His presence in the midst of your pain. Let's begin the healing journey . . .

———

"Yes, you're pregnant!"

Do you remember hearing those words or seeing the positive results from a test? What was your reaction? Your response to the news of expecting a child can be a lot like riding a roller coaster.

Some people respond with enthusiasm. They've longed to experience this ride and have anxiously awaited their turn. "Let's celebrate! We're finally on!" they shout. They race to the front of the roller coaster, ready to embrace the thrill of a lifetime.

Others hear the news and board the ride a bit cautious and reluctant. Seated a few rows from the front, they look nervous. They've been on the ride before but never made it to the end. Strapped in by fear and uncertainty, they cling to the hope that they'll complete the ride this time.

A third group of riders sits in the middle section of the coaster. They sport that in-between look—neither happy nor sad—as if they could take this ride or leave it. Some suspect these folks are in shock and don't believe it's true, perhaps because they've waited so long or never thought they'd get on the coaster at all.

At the back of the coaster sits another cluster of people. Like the first three groups, they are executives, home-makers, students, unemployed, married, single, young, old, rich, and poor. Jolted by the unexpected news or the loop-to-loop of their circumstances, they look as if they are about to get sick. Their solemn faces are powdered with disappointment, dread, and disbelief. "I can't believe I let this happen!" "I don't want a child!"

Maybe you can picture yourself in one of the groups. Although each of our circumstances, stories, and responses is different, most of you who hold this book share a common bond: never getting to the end of the ride, the pain of never fully knowing your child. Maybe you just started your journey, clicking up the track, and your coaster derailed when you were told, "Your levels are decreasing and you will miscarry," or "Your baby is growing outside your womb and emergency surgery is the only hope to save your life." Or were you well on your way to the end of the ride when your doctor told you the ride was over because "I cannot detect a heart-beat"? Did you perhaps make it to the end of the ride but shortly after your baby died? Or maybe you didn't want to be on the ride in the first place. A baby was not in your plans, and now your guilt for feeling that way is making you sick.

You have lost a child. So have I. Regardless of the circumstances, it's time to begin or continue the process of mending our broken hearts. Join me in the journey through grief as we face our loss together and invite God to guide us through.

Part 1

HIDING

Hiding: *to put out of sight; to conceal*
for shelter or protection; to keep secret

Rock of Ages, cleft for me,
Let me hide myself in Thee.

A. M. TOPLADY

My frame was not hidden from you
when I was made in the secret place,
when I was woven together in the depths of the earth.
Your eyes saw my unformed body;
all the days ordained for me were written in your book
before one of them came to be.

PSALM 139:15–16

Devotion 1

HIDE-AND-SEEK

*Then the man and his wife heard the sound of
the Lᴏʀᴅ God as he was walking in the garden in
the cool of the day, and they hid from the Lᴏʀᴅ
God among the trees of the garden. But the Lᴏʀᴅ
God called to the man, "Where are you?"*

Gᴇɴᴇsɪs 3:8–9

*H*ide-and-seek is one of my favorite childhood games.
I enjoy hiding. It's always a challenge to remain
silent and still when the seek-and-find mission is under
way. When footsteps tread close by and the person yells,
"Where are you?" I have to make a choice: Will I remain
hiding, or will I expose myself and be found?

That's the situation Adam and Eve found themselves
in after they disobeyed God and were hiding in the garden. I can only imagine the anguish they must have felt

when they realized that death was part of their lives now. They would experience death *physically* through the aging process, *emotionally* through guilt and shame, *socially* by blaming each other, and *spiritually* by alienating themselves from God because of sin. Picture this bereaved couple, mourning the lives they once had and peering out from the bushes, afraid they would be discovered and forced to face the truth.

Like Adam and Eve, you too have experienced a great loss. Whether through miscarriage, stillbirth, tubal pregnancy, or infant death, your loss may cause you to hide physically, emotionally, socially, or spiritually. Sometimes the pain is so intense that you may want to disconnect from others and from God. You look for ways to hide your hurt. You camouflage your questions, fears, and disappointment so well that you may think others do not notice. But how long can you stash your silent heartache? Is hiding really healthy, or does it hold you back from a healing journey? Sooner or later, someone will come to find you.

Do you find yourself hiding in the bushes like Adam and Eve? The Lord is walking through the garden, calling your name. How will you respond? Will you remain in hiding, or will you expose your real feelings about your loss and begin the journey through your grief?

God, the loss of my child is so agonizing. I feel as if I'm playing hide-and-seek with my pain. I've camouflaged my questions, fears, and hurts so that others will not notice and will pass me by. How long can I hide my heartache? Will You be my truth today? Reveal the specific areas of my life (physical, emotional, social, and spiritual) where I need healing. Show me how to move forward in my grief journey. Amen.

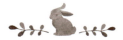

Steps Toward Healing

1. How have you been hiding the pain of your loss?

_____

_____

_____

_____

2. How have you felt disconnected physically? Emotionally? Socially? Spiritually?

_____

_____

_____

_____

_____

3. Imagine someone asking you, "Where are you
   in your grief?" How would you respond today? How
   would you like to respond a year from now?

_____

_____

_____

_____

_____

4. Are you ready now to take a few steps forward in
   grieving your child? If so, fill in the date below, and
   say this out loud.

   _Today, _____ (date), I am choosing not
   to hide my grief but to step forward in the journey to
   grieve my child._

Devotion 2

JOURNEY TO THE
HIDING PLACE

You are my hiding place;
you will protect me from trouble
and surround me with songs of deliverance.

PSALM 32:7

Sirens blare. The sky darkens. Trees rock frantically back and forth. The wind whirls violently. A funnel-shaped cloud descends. All are warning signs that a tornado is coming—and you'd better head for cover.

A tornado is a common occurrence in some parts of the United States. Its destructive wind has been known to demolish anything in its path: livestock, entire towns, and countless lives.

While growing up in Missouri, I learned that one of the safest places to be when a tornado hits is in the basement.

This below-ground-level room is a place where I weathered many storms and a few tornadoes. Whenever I scurried down the stairs to my hiding place, I felt safe. I had everything I needed: food, water, bedding, flashlights, a radio, a television, and games. Sometimes I even forgot about the storm because I couldn't see it or hear it.

Hidden below ground, unable to see or hear the storm, I could feel disconnected for minutes or hours. Only after the storm had passed and I ascended the stairs did I have to face the truth. On more than one occasion, what a shock it was to face reality! Broken tree limbs and debris blanketed our lawn. A pathway through town of uprooted trees and damaged power lines was a vivid reminder of the twister.

At times in your grief journey you may detect that a storm is coming. You may sense sirens blaring in your soul; your mood darkens or you feel frantic. Emotions whirl violently as the reality of your loss starts to descend upon you. It's time to head for cover. *To the basement!* you exclaim. You find yourself below the surface of reality, hiding from it. Your "basement" may be activity, exercise, or work. Maybe you hide by eating or curling up with a book. Your basement may look different from mine, but each of us has one—a place to hide. You don't have to face the questions, doubts, fears, and guilt. There are no people to respond to or excuses to make. Disconnected from reality, you may even forget about the storm of your loss.

But the pain of your loss hasn't gone away. With time, you must realize that you cannot live in the basement forever. When you finally ascend to face reality, you may be surprised to discover shattered dreams, a broken heart, emotional debris, uprooted expectations, and damaged relationships. But you will also find peace in knowing that the storm has passed.

Sure, you may have a lot of cleanup work to do, but there's unlimited eternal aid available. God will help you face the truth and will work with you to repair the damage. You can feel safe in His presence and in His Word. He wants to be the One to whom you run for shelter as you continue your journey. Will you let Him be your hiding place?

Lord, help! I'm hiding from the storm of my loss. I admit I've disconnected from reality by hiding my pain in _____. I need Your help to face the truth and to repair the damage that's been done in my life and in the lives of others. Come to my aid. Repair and restore my life. Remind me to run to Your presence and Your Word in my journey through grief. Be my hiding place and help me journey on. Amen.

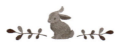

Steps Toward Healing

1. How do you hide from the storm of your loss?

_____

_____

_____

_____

_____

_____

2. Identify the emotional debris, uprooted expectations, or damaged relationships from your loss in need of repair. Write this in a prayer request to God.

_____

_____

_____

_____

_____

_____

3. Picture God as your hiding place. Read Psalm 32:8
   aloud as if God were responding to you today.
   Describe below what that looks and feels like.

_____

_____

_____

_____

_____

_____

Devotion 3

FACING THE TRUTH

Send out your light and your truth;
let them guide me.
Let them lead me to your holy mountain,
to the place where you live.

PSALM 43:3 NLT

ave you ever ignored the truth about your loss because reality was too painful to face? I have. For a season after my baby's death, coping with people and situations involving babies was challenging for me. I avoided certain activities, friends, restaurants, family, and even church on baby dedication day because I was afraid of how I would react. Making excuses worked for a while, but I realized I couldn't run from every situation and would have to find a way to survive.

One occasion happened a few months after our baby's death, when we traveled to spend Thanksgiving with family. I had conceived our child on the previous year's trip, which meant I would have to confront not only those memories, but also questioning stares, newborn babies, and those sporting maternity attire. During this trip, I had several "grief encounter moments" when I hid in the bathroom or mentally escaped.

Was this abnormal behavior? Some may think so. But looking back I realize that my seemingly irrational ways of coping were necessary for me at the time and enabled me to survive and to scale my mountain of grief. The story of a king and two mothers comes to mind.

Two women stood in front of King Solomon. One held a baby; the other clinged to an empty blanket. The woman with empty arms rushed forward and told Solomon about her son's birth. She choked back tears as she shared how the other woman gave birth to a son a few days later. But her baby died. This woman swapped the dead baby for the living baby while the new mother slept. "That's *my* baby," she moaned.

Silence pervaded the room. The king saw the pain in her eyes. He turned to face the woman holding the baby. She glared at him and shouted, "No, the living one is *my* son and the dead one is *hers*!"

What fear must have come into the heart of that baby's real mother. What boldness and denial were still in the heart of the mother whose child was dead.

Solomon commanded an attendant to bring him a sword. "Divide the living child in two, and give half to the one and half to the other."

"Oh, my lord, give her the living child and don't kill it," cried the woman with empty arms.

"Divide it!" said the other.

The truth couldn't be denied. The king, who was the wisest of judges, knew by the two mothers' words who was the real mother.

I can imagine how grateful that woman was as she reached for her baby and held him once again in her arms. Her tears turned to smiles, and the heaviness in her heart was replaced with joy.

But what about the other woman? Was she really cruelhearted and vindictive, or was she a desperate, grieving mother who would do anything to have her baby back?

What shock and pain this mother must have felt when she realized that her baby was dead. Did she convince herself he was only sleeping and would wake up soon? How tormenting for her to hear the other baby's healthy cry. No one would understand the anguish she felt. She couldn't face her loss. I wonder if she thought that just being near what she longed for would lessen her pain.

Perhaps, clutching her lifeless baby, she tiptoed into the room where everyone was sleeping. She bent down and peeked at the tiny breathing bundle. It felt so familiar. Maybe she thought, *I'll pick him up and hold him for just a few minutes.* She gently laid her baby down and scooped up the living baby into her arms. She didn't remember how long she held him or what happened next. All she knew was joy returned to her heart and a sense of relief that the death was just a terrible nightmare.

I'm not justifying or condoning this mother's actions. Yet I can relate to her pain and understand how grief can drive us to do, think, or say strange things. My brother and his wife had a healthy baby boy just a few days before my son was born and died. Although I was excited for them, the first few times I saw my nephew, he reminded me of what I longed for but didn't have. Sometimes when I held him, I would imagine that he was my son and allow myself to feel the joy of new motherhood, even if only for a few moments.

Through the years, I've watched my nephew grow into a bright, handsome, athletic young man who is about to graduate high school. He continues to be a sweet reminder to me of the age or stage my son would be. God used my nephew in my early years of grief to help me journey through denial, to fill my empty arms, comfort my grieving soul, and help me face the reality of my loss.

Fantasizing that your baby is still alive is one way to cope. Sometimes facing reality is too painful, and denying your loss is a temporary way to survive. In the right time, God will help you face reality and cope with your loss.

God, it feels like a dream that my child is gone, that I won't hear him or her crying, signaling that this is only a nightmare. My pain is too raw to face that reality right now. I want to pretend this never happened. It's like I'm standing in front of a judge with the truth on one side of me and denial on the other. You are the wise, discerning Judge, and You see my pain and the truth. Help me cope with the truth. Reveal it to me today. Amen.

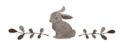

Steps Toward Healing

Read the story in 1 Kings 3:16–28.

1. Describe how each woman in the story responded
   to loss.

_____

_____

_____

_____

_____

_____

2. What would you say to each woman in the story?

_____

_____

_____

_____

_____

_____

3. How have you responded to others who have
   what you lost?

_____

_____

_____

_____

_____

_____

4. What would you like others to do for or say to you?

_____

_____

_____

_____

_____

_____

_____

Don't hide your pain. Be truthful with yourself, God,
and others this week. Seek the listening ear of a
person who is compassionate and trustworthy or has
experienced loss similar to yours.

Devotion 4

FROM MINIMIZING TO VALIDATING

You have searched me, Lord,
and you know me. . . .
My frame was not hidden from you
when I was made in the secret place.

PSALM 139:1, 15

"AT LEAST YOU LOST IT EARLY."
"You can always have another baby."
"Be thankful you have other children."
"You're so busy. Maybe it's for the best."
"You can always adopt."

Has anyone made a comment like this to you? If not, sooner or later a person might. These words were intended to comfort my husband and me after I miscarried our third baby a few weeks into my pregnancy. Instead, they intensified our pain by minimizing our loss. I'll never forget the devastating look in my husband's eyes when someone said, "Better to lose it now than later!" I was fuming inside and wanted to scream, *My baby was not an "it"! My baby was a person in the making, an individual just like you!*

Many people—family, friends, neighbors, coworkers, and the community—feel the trauma and tragedy of the death of adults and young lives. Obituaries validate their existence. But with a pregnancy loss, there are few memories, and the ones that exist live only for the woman and perhaps her husband. Who was this baby anyway? What was his identity? What contributions did she make to society? Many do not acknowledge a developing child as a viable life, and those who do may not understand why this type of individual was so significant and should be mourned.

How are we to grieve someone society does not expect us to grieve? Parents may mourn deeply, little, or not at all. There is no set mold or right way to mourn a loss. It is as normal for parents not to grieve as it is for them to be devastated. Those who mourn little or not at all initially may be minimizing their pain and may end up mourning the baby months or years later.

That's what happened to me after I miscarried our first child early in our marriage. Rich and I were having dinner with friends to celebrate his thirtieth birthday. We were excited that I was finally pregnant after years of trying. I excused myself to go to the bathroom. Moments later I knew I was losing our first child.

I resolved that I would not let this circumstance ruin Rich's celebration, so I resumed the party in progress as if nothing had happened. I quickly divorced myself from the disappointment of the miscarriage. I had a strong faith and assured the few friends who knew we had lost the baby that it was God's will and I was fine. I refused to mourn my loss. Instead, I minimized it and swept the sorrow of my loss under the rug of my smiles, activity, and work. Although I mouthed the words "I lost a child," their meaning didn't sink in until years later, after I suffered the death of our son and my third miscarriage.

Others who have not experienced losing a child probably won't understand how you feel or know how to respond to you. But your mourning does make sense. You lost a child. You have good reason to hurt. Don't minimize your pain! Pour out your heart to God. He understands. He is waiting with open arms to comfort you and validate the sorrow you've been hiding. He created your precious little one and knows your child by name. Let God embrace you with His love and compassion, just as He does your child in His heavenly kingdom.

Lord, should I really be feeling this way about losing my child? Am I making too much out of this loss? I know others don't understand how I feel. Help me to forgive the people who try to minimize my pain. My loss was a child, not an "it" or a mistake or a clump of cells. My child was part of me. You understand. You created my precious baby. It's comforting to know that You saw my child in my womb and know my child by name. My child has value in Your eyes. Give me courage to grieve and validate my pain. You are my Creator, the One who can form my loss into something good in time. Amen.

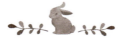

Steps Toward Healing

1. How have others minimized your loss? How does that make you feel? Why do you think others may have responded that way?

_____

_____

_____

_____

_____

2. Read Psalm 139 aloud. Which verses validate your
   child's worth? Circle or underline them. Write one of
   those verses here.

_____

_____

_____

_____

_____

3. People often make hurtful comments because they
   are uninformed. They may not fully understand that
   loss is loss and that you cannot compare how long
   you were pregnant or had a child to the level of grief
   you may feel. What could others say that would
   validate your loss?

_____

_____

_____

_____

_____

Devotion 5

MISSING IN ACTION

Be still, and know that I am God.

PSALM 46:10

Have you ever been so busy that you were unable to think or feel? I have.

Activity distracts me from facing the pain of my loss. In a sense, my to-do list keeps me missing in action. The more I do, the less I feel. The less I feel, the less I hurt. Hiding in my foxhole of busyness, I am sheltered from the battle zone of loss. I can avoid the cross fire of people's questions and the emotional explosions from my hurt. Armed with overcommitment and camouflaged by fatigue, I feel safe.

Unfortunately, I don't realize that I am at war with myself. Rest is my enemy. I convince myself that "busy is better," and the war inside me rages on. Then I'm hit with a missile of reality. It slows me down. I cringe in pain from the flashbacks of my losses.

Since most of my wounds from my loss aren't visible, I ignore them and keep moving. Then another missile of reality hits. My wound of fear is exposed. I'm afraid to face my loss. *Will I lose another child?* Control is my other unhealed battle scar. I couldn't control my body or the circumstances that led to the loss of my child, but I can control my schedule and how I grieve.

I need to heal, but I don't know how. Will I stay missing in action and delay the healing of my heart and soul, or will I come out of hiding and slow down to face the truth?

During a fourteen-month time frame, I lost an infant and had two miscarriages. I didn't realize that I was missing in action during that time in my life until I looked back at my calendar. My schedule was full. In addition to my job and my roles as wife and mother, I juggled more than twenty other roles. Whew! No wonder I was exhausted and didn't have time to think or feel.

Rest was nearly nonexistent. How could I expect myself to heal? At that time I didn't even know that I needed to. I thought I was doing fine and handling my grief in a positive manner. I didn't even realize I needed to slow down until I attended a weekend retreat in the mountains.

Cool air and pine trees replaced my phone and the Internet. One of the planned activities during the weekend was to spend time alone with God. I plopped down beneath a tree by a rushing stream. Then a missile of reality hit my soul: *Be still, and know that I am God.*

I began to weep. Then another missile hit, this time exposing the wounds of my loss: *Cast all your cares on Me, because I care for you* (1 Peter 5:7).

For the first time in a long time, I had uninterrupted time with God. I poured out my heart to Him about the pain of my loss and my need for Him to help me slow down. That was a defining moment in my journey through grief. I finally acknowledged and faced the pain of the loss I'd been hiding in my activity. I was ready to journey on.

Are you missing in action and unable to heal the wounds from your loss? Have you allowed your activity to replace your sensitivity to your pain? Are you at war with yourself? Maybe it's time to slow down and escape from your busyness.

That's what Jesus did after He suffered the loss of His cousin John the Baptist. He released His activity and went away to a lonely place to spend time with God. Learn from His example. Stop hiding in activity. Be still in God's presence. It's a necessary stop in your grief journey.

> Lord, please help me slow down! I'm missing in action. My schedule is so busy that I don't have time to think or feel. Am I hiding in the foxhole of busyness to avoid the battle zone of my loss? Let a missile of reality through Your Word hit my soul. Expose the wounds from my loss, and heal them. You are the Victor. Bring peace to the war within my soul so I can journey on. Amen.

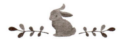

Steps Toward Healing

1. Are you too busy? Make a list of your roles and the activities associated with each role during a typical week. Is time alone with God on your list?

_____

_____

_____

_____

_____

2. Do you feel as if you've been avoiding facing your
   hurt? Why or why not? Why do you think it is so
   difficult for you to be still?

_____

_____

_____

_____

_____

3. Where is your "foxhole of faith," the physical
   place where you go to be still with God? If you don't
   have a place, where could you go? Read Psalm 46;
   Matthew 11:28; and Psalm 5.

_____

_____

_____

_____

_____

_____

4. Schedule at least ten minutes each day to be still with God. Take your list of activities to Him and ask Him to show you the roles you need to release for a time.

5. Are there others who can help you face reality and share your load? Who are they?

_____

_____

_____

_____

_____

_____

Part 2

SUFFERING

Suffering: *to endure*
hardship or suffer loss

CHILDREN'S FOOTPRINTS

Some children come into our lives and go quickly.
Some children come into our lives and stay awhile.
All our children come into our lives and leave footprints—
Some oh so small;
Some a little larger;
Some, larger still,
But all have left their footprints on our lives; in our hearts,
And we will never, never be the same.

DOREEN SEXTON

Devotion 6

NOTHING TO SHOW
FOR MY LOSS

Where does understanding dwell? . . .
God understands the way to it
and he alone knows where it dwells.

JOB 28:20, 23

W hen you lose a child, you feel a poignant pain. Your dream of experiencing your child develop, be born, and grow up is snatched away. And you may feel as if you have nothing to show for your loss but a stack of bills, an out-of-shape body, raging hormones, an incomplete nursery, pain and suffering, and empty arms. It doesn't seem fair. But we live in a fallen world, and the pain and suffering of that world touches our lives too. Nothing will be totally fair and perfect until we get to heaven.

Since our world is fallen, we are all victims of heartache at one time or another. Your miscarriage, stillbirth, tubal pregnancy, or infant loss isn't a sign of sin in your life or a message from God to "clean up your act." It is simply a form of suffering common to the human experience of living in this world.

When we discovered in the fourth month of my pregnancy with John Samuel that he had a fatal defect and would die unless God performed a miracle, I plummeted to a new depth of suffering. I believed God could heal our son and proclaimed this publicly to others. I also predetermined that if He chose not to heal our son, I would praise God anyway.

During the months that followed, I endured the skeptical looks of those who thought I was in denial and the pain of being ignored by others. Most days were bittersweet. I cherished every moment my son kicked and the hours he kept me up at night. I talked to him, read to him, and prayed aloud for him. I knew that as long as he was in my womb, he was safe and alive.

When I entered the hospital at forty-two weeks to be induced, I hoped God would answer our prayer and I would bring our healthy, healed baby home. During the long, intense labor, I suffered the pain of uncertainty, not knowing if my child would live or die. It wasn't until my son was born and the doctor placed him in my arms that I knew I would have to say "hello" and then "good-bye."

The reality of this suffering didn't impact me until I was alone and looked down at my stomach. I realized John Samuel was gone—and I had nothing to show for my labor or his life except an expanded waistline and a limp blanket. The next day, when my husband wheeled me out of the hospital, I felt awkward and empty. My heart ached with certainty, knowing my son was with Jesus, but my arms were empty.

Jesus understands your journey through suffering. In the Garden of Gethsemane, He pleaded with God to take His cup of suffering from Him. But He willingly offered to accept His suffering if that was part of God's plan. He suffered rejection from His friends, physical and emotional abuse, public humiliation, cruel comments, physical torture, and death on a cross. Did He deserve it? No. He was innocent. Yet Jesus knew that our world is fallen and that there was no hope to redeem humanity's spiritual suffering but for Him to die on the cross for our sins.

What if you were to ask Jesus' mother, Mary, "What do you have to show for the loss of your Son?" She might reply, "Empty arms and the assurance of living eternally with my Son, Jesus, in heaven." That's the good news about suffering. Jesus has "been there, done that." He can relate to what you're experiencing, but He wants to give you hope to see your loss in the scope of eternity. He is willing to take your cup of suffering and walk with you through your pain. Go ahead—give Him your cup of suffering now. Allow Him to fill your arms with His hope and salvation.

God, my arms are empty. I have nothing to show for my loss, and it seems so unfair. I didn't expect things to turn out this way. You could have saved my child, but You didn't. You are the One who understands and sees the big picture, even if I don't. Please take my cup of suffering, and walk with me through my pain. Wrap Your arms of understanding and comfort around me. Fill my empty arms with Your hope and salvation. Amen.

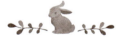

Steps Toward Healing

1. Recall the first time after you lost your child when you realized you had empty arms. What emotions did you encounter?

_____

_____

_____

_____

_____

2. Some women who have lost children say that "aching arms" is a common occurrence and that holding something helps ease the pain. What could you hold?

_____

_____

_____

_____

_____

3. Jesus was innocent, yet He willingly suffered and died. How does His example give you hope?

_____

_____

_____

_____

Journey Through the Darkness of Depression

But you, LORD, do not be far from me.
You are my strength; come quickly to help me.

PSALM 22:19

Tracy sat in her office, unable to concentrate. She couldn't complete her work regardless of how hard she tried. Over the past several months since losing her baby, careless mistakes and a negative and critical attitude were the norm for her. Exhaustion and a loss of appetite were her constant companions. Her generally positive outlook about people and life had faded.

One morning Tracy couldn't get out of bed. She felt as if all the electricity in her life had been shut off and darkness was closing in. Fear gripped her. She felt so out of control and lost. What was happening to her? She had a strong faith and supportive family and friends. Known for her optimism and reliance on God, Tracy was the model of physical and spiritual health. But at that moment, Tracy felt weak and alone. She knew something was terribly wrong, but she didn't know how to overcome this personal power outage in her life. She was afraid of what others would think if she cried out for help.

The darkness of depression is common in the journey through grief. Like Tracy, you may be trekking along your lighted path of life and appear unaffected by your loss. You've acknowledged your loss, allowed yourself to grieve, talked about it, gone to support groups, and read Scripture. Maybe you haven't noticed that your attitude, appetite, or ability to cope with everyday activities has dimmed and is getting darker.

Even if you are aware of the changes in your life, you may choose to make excuses or rationalize them away rather than face the darkness of depression that may be closing in. *Good Christians shouldn't struggle with depression,* you think. *Maybe I'm just working too hard or need to exercise more than I am. I know my baby is with God, so I should feel relieved and glad.*

The darkness of depression can occur at any time

during your grief journey. It may hit suddenly and severely, like "lights out" in a power outage during a storm, or it may be more gradual, like a dimmer on your light switch. Or you may be one of the fortunate ones who never or only moderately encounters depression.

I used to cringe if someone would ask me, "Kathe, are you depressed?" I felt as if depression meant I was weak or incompetent in some way. "It's probably my hormones," I rationalized. "I'm writing this book, which is really painful." It wasn't until a well-known Christian leader who had also lost a child told me about her depression that I accepted that my angry outbursts, cluttered home, inability to finish projects, forgetfulness, frequent tears, and negative attitude could all be symptoms of depression.

In the dark night of my soul, I discovered I was not alone. David penned many of his psalms when he was depressed. Hannah wept and was deeply distressed because she desired a child.

Facing the darkness and seeking medical or professional expertise to help you journey through depression is often necessary. God wants to be the light to guide us through. Often in our blackest moments, we discover that His light shines brightest. Ask Him to guide you to others who can help illuminate your path so you can journey on.

God, darkness is closing in on my life. I can't cope with life the way I used to. I need Your help! Help me face my pain. Restore me. Be my light, and guide me through the dark night of my soul. Guide me to others who can illuminate my path and help me journey through. Amen.

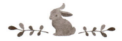

Steps Toward Healing

1. In what specific ways are you having difficulty coping with life?

_____

_____

_____

_____

_____

2. What steps can you take to seek help?

_____

_____

_____

_____

_____

3. Whom do you know who could brighten your path and
   help you journey through the dark night of your soul?

_____

_____

_____

_____

_____

THE EMPTY FRAME

If we had forgotten the name of our God
or spread out our hands to a foreign god,
would not God have discovered it,
since he knows the secrets of the heart?

PSALM 44:20–21

$\mathcal{P}$am discovered she was pregnant, but before she could share her news with her boyfriend, she lost the baby. *No one needs to know what happened!* she rationalized to herself. Locked in a hidden safe behind the picture of her life was her secret. She didn't want to disappoint her parents, so she vowed never to tell them.

Life continued for Pam. She graduated from college, started a career, married, and had two children. She forgot about the child she'd lost, or so she thought—until one Thanksgiving.

Pam always looked forward to large family gatherings at her mom's. "Going home" for Thanksgiving was the one tradition that everyone in her family kept. She could hardly wait to see how much her nieces and nephews had grown since last year.

"We're here!" Pam's children announced as they scurried up the front steps and gave their grandmother a hug. Pam walked inside. The aromas of fresh-baked bread and apple pie filled the air. *Mom still remembers my favorites.* Memories of growing up there flooded her mind. She strolled into the living room and spied the old piano. *I wonder if I still remember how to play*, she thought as she sat down and placed her fingers on the ivory keys. To her amazement, she did. She struck the final chord and looked up with a confident glow. An audience of framed photographs atop the piano stared back at her.

Pictures of grandchildren were among her mother's most valued possessions, which she displayed proudly. Pictures were *another* tradition. Pam marveled at how her children had changed through the years. She chuckled at the grandchildren's group shot taken last year: "Five Pilgrims and Five Indians." *But there should be one more*, Pam thought. Tears stung her eyes. *My child would be the oldest grandchild. But no one knows my child*

GRIEVING THE *Child* I NEVER KNEW

is missing. My child never had a name. Why didn't I tell anyone?

I'm the only one who knows the combination to the safe that hides my secret. Should I open the door and tell my family? What would they think now? Or should I keep my secret locked away?

Then Pam saw an empty wooden picture frame on the piano. She picked it up and held it for a while, then set it down again. *I wonder what my child would look like. Would he have my eyes? In time, maybe I'll share my secret. For now, I'll just tuck my secret back inside and silently remember him every time I look at the empty frame.*

Sometimes you may grieve in private. Did you keep your pregnancy a secret because you were afraid or unsure how people might react? Maybe you thought it wasn't a big deal if you lost your child in the first few weeks. Or was it too painful to share about your loss because it made you feel like a failure? Even if others do know about your loss, at times they may forget to acknowledge your child or include him in the "count" of children or grandchildren.

If you talk about your child openly, do others seem uncomfortable? Maybe that's why you've chosen to be silent. But your heart yearns to speak your child's name, if your child had one. So what if your child is nameless? It's never too late to give a name. I named each of the children I miscarried, sometimes years after the actual loss occurred.

Even though I was unsure about their genders, I sensed that they were boys. Naming my children helped me validate them as individuals and relieve some of my pain and uncertainty about their identity. Although some people raise their eyebrows when I call the children I lost by name, framing their existence with names helps me honor them and relate to them, even if I never knew them.

How have you been suffering in secret? What are you hiding in the safe behind the picture of your life? God knows the combination to your personal safe. Maybe it's time to let Him open the door to expose the secret suffering of your loss. Is there an empty picture frame inside? What does it represent to you? Your child is precious to God, and He knows your child by name, even if you or others do not.

Naming your child may be a healing process for you. You may share it with others or only whisper it to yourself. That's up to you. If you choose not to name your child, that's okay too. What's important is to know that God loves you and is here to journey with you through the secret places of your life. He is all-knowing and will never forget you or the child you lost. You are framed forever in His heart.

God, You know the secrets I have locked away in my heart. I feel as if I can't say my child's name or share my true feelings with others because they won't understand. So I suffer in secret. Sometimes I try to hide my suffering from You too. But I can't. You know exactly what I'm feeling. Open the door to my loss, and help me look inside. Fill the empty picture frame of my loss with Your acceptance and compassion. Amen.

Steps Toward Healing

1. How have you suffered in secret about your loss?

_____

_____

_____

_____

_____

_____

_____

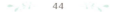

2. What feelings have you locked away?

_____

_____

_____

_____

_____

3. Describe your empty picture frame. How do you feel when you look at it?

_____

_____

_____

_____

_____

4. Naming your child is not necessary, but it is certainly acceptable to God. If you did not name your child and would like to, do so now.

_____

_____

_____

_____

HAPPY-SAD DAYS

"I the Lord do not change."

Malachi 3:6

"Mommy, why do you look so sad today?" My young son's question startled me as I glanced at myself in the rearview mirror.

I do look sad, I thought. *But why?* I checked off each item from my mental list:

- hormones
- time of month
- lack of sleep
- caffeine

- anniversary date of my baby's death
- day of the week

No, it wasn't any of these.

"I don't know, Jake," I responded. My answer seemed to appease him, but it sparked my curiosity. I was determined to solve the mystery behind my feelings.

Mood swings, tears, and depression had been familiar companions since losing my baby. I never knew when they would appear at the doorstep of my emotions, though often a holiday, event, or memory summoned their presence. I recall one Mother's Day at church, when all the women who had babies that year were asked to stand. I remained seated, but I wanted to stand and scream, "I had a baby too!"

The day I received free baby products and a coupon for a baby portrait in the mail, I erupted into tears. The day of Jake's first-grade open house was a tender time when his teacher showed me his family sketch: three stick figures holding hands in front of a house and stick figures in the clouds.

Lord, what is triggering my emotions today? I prayed silently. *Help me label my unnamed suffering.* Then it hit me. *It's my due date! I should be in labor today and celebrating the arrival of my precious baby. How could I have forgotten?* Guilt knocked at my heart's door, but I refused to let it in.

Instead, I gave myself permission to think about the child I never knew. *What would he look like? What would his cry sound like? How would it feel to hold him? Would he enjoy baths? How would he and his brother get along?*

I continued to ponder. *Does he know that I almost forgot about today? Does he know that I love him and miss him? What is it like for him to be in God's presence and to have no suffering?*

Suddenly I realized that Jake was staring at me. "Mom, why do you look *mostly* happy now?"

"Well, I'm happy today because our baby is in heaven, but I'm sad because he would have been born today." I could tell by my son's silence that he was pondering my comment as we waited at the red light.

Then Jake shouted, "Mom, it's like being a yellow light . . . You're not red and you're not green, but you're a little of each!" Jake squeezed my arm and our eyes locked. Amazingly, God used a child and a traffic signal to reveal the truth and affirm my happy-sad emotions that day.

Maybe it's time for you to review your list of holidays, events, or memories. You may discover that today is significant and you have just cause to feel the way you do. Or today may just be a typical day and you feel deeply for no apparent reason. That's possible, too, of course.

Grief *is* a lot like a traffic signal—you never know

how long it will last or whether you'll feel happy or sad or somewhere in between on a certain day. And just when you think you've figured it out, it changes.

Lord, what is triggering my emotions today? Is today a significant day? Some of my memories make me smile, and others make me sad. I know that it's okay for me to feel both emotions at the same time. Even though my feelings change frequently like a traffic signal, You never do. Your truth is constant. Every day is significant because You are there. Gently remind me of Your presence in my pain, and show me how to make it count for good. Amen.

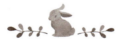

Steps Toward Healing

1. Take a few moments to reflect on your child. How old would he or she be now? What do you think he or she would be like?

_____

_____

_____

_____

_____

2. Certain dates may trigger happy-sad emotions about your child. Some people may grieve these dates silently, while others find it helpful to express their grief through planting a tree or giving to a special cause in memory of their child. What is your plan?

_____

_____

_____

_____

_____

3. Write a letter to your child in heaven. Ask questions. Share your feelings.

_____

_____

_____

_____

_____

Devotion 10

HUSBANDS AND WIVES
GRIEVE DIFFERENTLY

"Blessed are those who mourn,
for they will be comforted."

MATTHEW 5:4

Hannah and her husband, Elkanah, were a godly Israelite couple in the Bible who enjoyed a loving marriage. When Hannah wept over her barrenness, her husband tried his best to comfort her: "Hannah, why are you weeping? Why don't you eat? Why are you downhearted? Don't I mean more to you than ten sons?" (1 Samuel 1:8).

I can only imagine how Hannah must have felt when she heard his words. Although she knew her husband loved her, his words must have cut to the core of her being. Did

Hannah feel as if she were standing on one side of the Grand Canyon and her husband were on the other with the canyon of loss between them?

Elkanah was her best friend. She had always been able to talk to him about anything, and he had always affirmed her feelings. That was one of the qualities she admired most about him. She didn't expect *him* to say such cold and unfeeling words. Did Hannah look at Elkanah in that moment and see him more as a distant stranger? How empty and alone she must have felt. Disappointment must have overwhelmed her when she realized her handsome prince was really a frog when it came to understanding her feelings. Why couldn't he understand her pain, see through her eyes, and feel the ache in her soul each time she saw a pregnant woman or baby?

How Hannah must have longed for Elkanah to wrap his arms around her and say, "Honey, I'm so sorry you're hurting. I feel the same way." Instead, he tried to minimize her pain. Did he really believe he could make up for her loss and satisfy all her desires? Every time he gave her that knowing look in their bedroom, did she feel inadequate and less of a woman? The pain of desiring a child was enough to endure, but now she had to cope with the loss of his understanding too.

Loss often reveals the distance that can exist between two loving people. You and your husband may express sorrow differently. Women tend to talk openly about their pain and express emotions, while some men appear cold and unfeeling and sometimes spend more time away from home by losing themselves in work.

You may feel as if your husband is uncaring and doesn't understand your grief. Most men cannot talk easily about their pain and may express grief only when alone. Because men don't bond with the unborn baby the same way women do, men usually grieve differently. I realized this a few days after my third miscarriage when I asked my husband how he felt about the loss of our child. He shrugged his shoulders, gave me his analytical engineer look, and said, "I don't feel anything. I don't think of our loss as losing a child since I never saw the child or related to him."

Ouch! His words hurt. For a moment I felt as if Rich were on one side of the Grand Canyon and I was on the other. How we felt about our child and our loss was the chasm separating us. How I longed to remove the distance I was experiencing. I wanted him to understand the emptiness and sorrow I felt. How I wished I could wave my magic wand and transform his understanding to be like mine.

But I couldn't. God created Rich different from me. Rich, like most men, is a competitive problem solver. He sees himself in the role of protector. He experienced the pregnancy through me—that was his only connection to our unborn child. Since most men are result oriented, they may consider a person as someone they can touch and feel, which in most cases may not be an unborn child. "To me it was just a cluster of cells," one father said, "but to [my wife] it was a little boy."

Men often seek comfort from their loss through physical intimacy. Physical intimacy can ease a man's emotional pain. Sometimes the bedroom may become a battleground if you do not understand the way your partner grieves. You may view your bedroom as the place where your child was conceived, and it may be painful for you. When your husband gives you that knowing look, you may be thinking, *You want to do* what? *It's only been a short time since we lost our child!* You may feel as if your husband is being thoughtless and distant, when in reality he is trying to close the emotional gap he is feeling.

Your husband speaks a different grief language than you do. You may need to ask him to translate what comforts him or what he needs. And be prepared to do the same. Often I just need to talk about it, but I don't want Rich to minimize my pain or try to solve the problem. I've learned to be direct and tell my husband how I need him to support me in my grief. When I say, "I don't need you to solve my problem; I just need you to listen," he is relieved and usually understands.

Your journey through grief is different from your husband's. At times, you may feel misunderstood and suffer alone. But you are not alone. God is there with you, and He understands your pain and suffering. He knows what you are thinking and feeling before you ever say a word. And He understands your husband too. He knows how difficult it is for your husband to see you in pain. Ask God to help you see past hurtful comments and actions from a father who has lost a child too and who doesn't know how to solve the problem for his wife.

God, I feel so alone in my suffering. I wish my husband could understand exactly how I feel, but he can't. I know he loves me, but sometimes I look at him as if he's a stranger. At times, his words and actions meant to comfort me only make my pain worse. Forgive me for the way I feel and for wrong actions and words I've spoken to him. Be my Communicator. Translate my words and actions to my husband. Help me be sensitive to him. Transform my hurt to hope and the distance I feel to a deepened relationship with You. Amen.

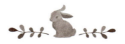

Steps Toward Healing

1. God created you and your spouse to be different and unique. How do each of you express grief differently?

_____

_____

_____

_____

_____

_____

2. How has your loss created distance between you and your spouse? Drawn you closer?

_____

_____

_____

_____

_____

_____

3. Complete the following sentence: "I feel loved and encouraged when . . ." Write down all the ways you feel loved and encouraged, and ask your spouse to do the same. Then exchange lists and encourage each other during the next week.

_____

_____

_____

_____

_____

4. Grief over the loss of your child will affect your relationship. Some marriages may become weakened from the stress while others are strengthened as the partners pull together through adversity. Guard your marriage and seek help from your pastor, another couple who has survived the loss of a child, or a grief counselor. What is your plan?

_____

_____

_____

_____

_____

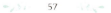

Part 3

QUESTIONING

Questioning: *to cross-examine, doubt, dispute, examine, analyze, inquire*

Clearly unless the Lord chooses to explain Himself to us, which often He does not, . . . many of our questions—especially those that begin with the word why—*will have to remain unanswered for the time being.*
Dr. James Dobson, *When God Doesn't Make Sense*

As you do not know the path of the wind, or how the body is formed in a mother's womb, so you cannot understand the work of God, the Maker of all things.
Ecclesiastes 11:5

DROWNING IN
THE SEA OF WHY

"When you pass through the waters,
I will be with you;
and when you pass through the rivers,
they will not sweep over you."

ISAIAH 43:2

*M*ommy, why do all our babies have to die?"
This question still left me speechless, though it was not the first time my son had asked it. Should I respond differently than I had before to my brokenhearted son, who had prayed fervently for a baby?

At that moment I felt as if I had just been thrown overboard and was drowning in the Sea of Why. I too had questions that flooded my mind. Why, after we suffered a miscarriage and adopted Jake, did our baby, John

Samuel, die? Why, after losing him, did I have two more miscarriages? And why was my son still asking me the same question?

The Sea of Why was massive and encircled me. Waves of wondering crashed against my soul. The undercurrent of uncertainty began to pull me beneath the dark, mysterious surface. I struggled to stay afloat, but it seemed the more I questioned, the deeper I sank into the unknown. *God, please help me!* I prayed. *I don't know what to say to my son this time.*

Suddenly, my spirit buoyed. *That's it!* I thought. I sensed God's answer as He revealed the line of hope that would rescue me. "I still don't know, Jake," I said as I gazed deep into his eyes. "All I know is that God is there, He is good, and that's enough." I felt relieved to admit to myself once again, *God, I don't understand!*

Often we don't understand the whys of our circumstances. Our questions remain unanswered, and we find ourselves flailing in the Sea of Why. What we believe about God during those times of uncertainty will influence how we respond. If we believe that our circumstance is something Satan slipped by God when He wasn't looking, we will plummet to the depths and drown in despair. But if we view the God of the Bible as sovereign, supreme, and the One who calms the waters, we will be buoyed with hope.

We will see purpose, even though we may not know now what the purpose is.

Most of us in the journey of grieving the child we never knew will find ourselves in the Sea of Why, pondering our loss. During times of questioning, I reflect on Job's life and remember that God allows suffering and has purpose in our pain. I must choose to look beyond the *why* and to the *Who* and view my loss through the lens of God rather than human sight.

Are you drowning in the Sea of Why? God understands. He is there. He is good. Look to Him. Sometimes that's the only answer there is.

> God, even though I still don't understand why this has happened and maybe never will, I know that You are unchanging, trustworthy, in control, and good. I believe You have a purpose for what has taken place. Forgive me for asking the same questions. Buoy me up once again with Your hope and truth. As I continue to journey through questioning, rescue me from drowning in despair. Help me trust You with all my heart and not lean on my own understanding. Give me divine vision, and enable me to see beyond the *why* and to the *Who*. Amen.

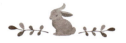

Steps Toward Healing

1. What questions about your loss remain unanswered?

_____

_____

_____

_____

_____

_____

2. Are there resources, people, or professionals who
   may have answers? What steps could you take to
   seek solutions?

_____

_____

_____

_____

_____

_____

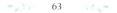

3. Like Job, we may never have our questions answered. How does that make you feel? It's interesting to note in the book of Job that, in response to sixteen *why*s, there are fifty-nine *who*s, which refer to God. The next time you ask *Why?* about your loss, consider changing the *y* in that word to an *o*.

_____

_____

_____

_____

_____

Devotion 12

WHY AM I SO ANGRY?

Get rid of all bitterness, rage and anger.

Ephesians 4:31

*P*aul slammed the door. Sara knew by the way her husband stomped up the steps after talking to their neighbors that he was angry.

"What's wrong?" she asked.

"Judy's pregnant!" he snapped. "She told me she didn't even want to have a third child. It was an accident."

Sara could see behind her husband's anger to the hurt and disappointment he felt as he blurted out, "We've been trying to have a child for nearly two years, and all we have to show for it is temperature charts, ovulation kits, and a positive pregnancy stick before we lost the baby. Why her and not us?"

Jennie thought the family reunion would lift her spirits. This was her first public outing since losing her second stillborn son. The doctor could not determine the cause of death and warned her not to have another child. Plagued with sorrow, she did her best to enjoy conversation, food, and games with her relatives.

Everything was going fine until her sister-in-law approached her with a baby in her arms. She felt as if the dam was about to break on her emotions, though somehow she managed to hold them back until she arrived home. Then she released the floodgate of tears and anger. *Why did I lose my sons? Why was my sister-in-law so insensitive? Why can't I have a baby like she did? If God is so good, why did He allow this to happen to me?*

For years Jennie had made excuses about why she avoided her sister-in-law and didn't like her. Her unanswered stream of questions about her loss was now a raging river of anger. Unaware that she had allowed her hostility to build and separate her from others, Jennie finally realized that she needed to face her dam of anger and discover how she could release it as well.

Anger is a natural part of the grieving process. Of all the grieving responses, I believe anger is the most difficult to accept, especially if you are a Christian. You may feel angry at your spouse, who did not support you in the way you wanted, or at friends, for things they said. Perhaps you are mad at other women who have complication-free pregnancies and give birth to healthy babies. Or perhaps you are furious at women who have aborted a child.

Maybe you've shouted at your body, "Why did you let me down?" You may find you get angry at little things that never used to bother you. And if you are honest enough to admit it, you might even be angry at God. Have you ever wanted to scream, "God, You have the power of life and death. You could have performed a miracle and protected my baby, yet You didn't! Why?"

For a long time, anger scared me. I didn't feel it was an appropriate response to my pain. It wasn't until a friend challenged me to write a letter to God and share my personal disappointments that I realized how dammed up my anger had become. As I sat alone in my backyard with a blank notebook and pen in my hand, I released my floodgate of questions and emotions. Several red-penned pages later, I felt as if the waters of my life were flowing peacefully.

Since then, I've learned that anger is a natural, necessary part of the journey through grief. Anger is usually a secondary emotion blocking the real cause of our pain. It may be disguised as rejection, disappointment, unmet expectations, envy, guilt, fear, or a multitude of other possibilities. When I feel angry, I stop and ask myself, "*Why* am I angry? *What* is behind the anger I feel?"

Your journey through anger can be healthy, healing, and righteous. Open the Bible: God, Moses, Job, the authors of the Psalms, and the prophets all demonstrate righteous anger. Jesus Himself overturned the tables of the money changers in the temple.

Conflicts between men, women, and God have existed since Adam and Eve ate the forbidden fruit in the garden of Eden. So why should you feel so uncomfortable about your anger? When restoration and peace occur in our walk with God, it is often after a floodgate release of anger. In the personal history of many Christians, a holy outburst or revolt has been the first step toward a trusting encounter with God.

Do you or others you know feel angry? If so, that's okay. God created anger, and He gives you permission to express yourself in a healthy, righteous way. But *why* are you angry? *What's* behind the anger you feel? Did someone disappoint you with the way he or she responded to your loss? Are you envious of others who have what you desire? Are you mad at yourself and feeling guilty or afraid? Or do you believe that God let you down and rejected your pleas for help?

Maybe it's time to face the anger you've dammed up. Tell God what has disappointed you. Ask Him to show you the truth and the real cause behind the dam of anger you have allowed to build. God wants to help you release it and open up the floodgate so that you are restored and the river of your life is flowing peacefully in Him.

God, why do I feel so angry? Anger scares me. It makes me feel uncomfortable. What is really behind the anger I feel? Reveal my disappointments. Please show me how to have righteous anger. Break down the dam of anger I've allowed to separate me from others and from You. Open the floodgates, and let the river of Your truth flow through my life so that I am restored and have peace. Amen.

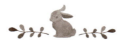

Steps Toward Healing

1. How have you recently expressed healthy, righteous anger over your loss? Unhealthy anger?

_____

_____

_____

_____

_____

_____

2. What do you feel is behind your anger? Disappointment? Envy? Expectations? Guilt? Physical exhaustion? Fear? Rejection?

_____

_____

_____

_____

_____

_____

3. Tell God how you feel. Write a letter to Him and
   share your heart.

_____

_____

_____

_____

_____

_____

_____

_____

_____

_____

_____

_____

_____

_____

_____

_____

_____

_____

_____

_____

Devotion 13

WHY DO I
FEEL SO GUILTY?

*My guilt has overwhelmed me like
a burden too heavy to bear.*

PSALM 38:4

$\mathcal{A}$fter the birth of Jesus, King Herod ordered all male children under three years of age in Bethlehem to be killed. The Bible says you could hear weeping and mourning throughout the entire city. I'm sure the grieving chorus included parents, grandparents, brothers, sisters, aunts, uncles, cousins, friends, and neighbors.

I can only imagine the gut-wrenching shock and horror the parents must have felt when their precious children were seized from them against their will. *This can't be happening! There must be some mistake! I'll do anything you ask to save my child!* Despite their protests, pleas, and prayers, they were unable to protect their children. How helpless and anguished these parents must have felt. *I should have tried harder to save my child. There must have been something I could have done. Why didn't I leave town? I failed.* Did the weight of guilt nearly crush them?

Guilt is one of the most common and intense feelings after the loss of your child. It's a normal part of your grief journey. It is common to wonder if you did something to cause this or if you could have prevented your child's death.

You may spend hours going over your actions during your pregnancy or in the days before the baby died. *Did I do everything the doctor said? Did I eat right and rest? Was my stress level too high? Were the medications or tests responsible for my loss? Should I have gone to a different doctor or had more tests? Was sexual activity the cause? Would more bed rest have helped?*

Don't punish yourself by replaying your past to figure out if you could have done something differently. If the "what ifs" and "if onlys" keep plaguing you for too long, they can damage your self-confidence and your relationships.

Maybe it's time to press Stop and focus on the One who understands your suffering and can free you from your guilt. Did you know that no suffering can touch you without having first received the permission of God? God is sovereign. He allowed the Bethlehem slayings, and He allowed your child to die. As painful as this truth may be to face, sooner or later, you must. No one can fully explain God's actions or plans but God.

As you journey through questioning, remember that guilt is not intended to drive you from God but toward Him. He sees beyond where you are today and will help you press Play and move forward. Will you let Him today?

God, I feel as if I could have done something to save my child. It's hard for me to accept that it's not my fault. I keep replaying my pregnancy in my mind. Please help me to hit Stop and look to You. You are the answer. You are sovereign. Nothing can touch my life without Your permission. Help me stop blaming myself. When I feel guilty, remind me to run to You. Help me press Play today and move forward. Amen.

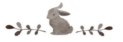

Steps Toward Healing

1. How have you blamed yourself for losing your child?

_____

_____

_____

_____

_____

_____

2. Read aloud Isaiah 46:9–10; Matthew 10:29–30; and 2 Chronicles 20:6. God is sovereign. He has supreme authority and power. He controls everything. How does this truth change your perspective?

_____

_____

_____

_____

_____

_____

3. Write the previous verses on three-by-five-inch cards. When you sense that you are replaying the guilt from your loss, stop . . . then look at the truth.

Devotion 14

GOD, WHERE ARE YOU?

Do not be afraid; do not be discouraged, for the
Lord your God will be with you wherever you go.

JOSHUA 1:9

Martha looked worried. She had never seen her brother, Lazarus, so sick before. He was so weak that he could barely walk, and now he was refusing to eat. All of the home remedies she had tried weren't working. And the local doctors just shook their heads. *What more can I do to help him?* she thought.

Then it occurred to her to contact their good friend Jesus. He was a frequent guest in their home and knew Lazarus well. He was known for helping and healing the sick, so much so that one of His nicknames was "the Healer." He would know what to do. Martha sent word to Jesus, requesting His immediate assistance. She felt confident Jesus would come to her aid and heal Lazarus.

She expected Jesus to arrive at their home at any moment, but He didn't. *Where are You?* Martha wondered. This wasn't like the Jesus she thought she knew. He was usually quick to respond. She couldn't understand why He hadn't at least acknowledged her request and sent a return message. Martha felt He had abandoned her at a time when she needed Him most. With each passing day, Martha's hopes faded. Finally it was too late. Lazarus died.

Maybe you can relate to Martha. Did you cry out for God to save your child, believing He would? Did you ask Him to come near, but He kept you waiting and wondering? Do you feel as if God gave you the silent treatment and didn't respond in the way or in the timing you thought He should have?

When I am on the phone with a friend, I expect her to answer me when I ask her a question. When I wait for a response and hear silence, I begin to wonder if we have been disconnected or if my friend has hung up on me or if maybe she wasn't paying attention. Silence may mean she is no longer on the line, but it may also mean she is waiting to respond. Sometimes I instinctively know my friend is still on the line even though there is silence. I may not understand the delay or the timing in which she answers me, but she is still on the line and she is still my friend.

When Jesus finally arrived after Lazarus had been dead for four days, Martha confronted Him: "Lord . . . if you had been here, my brother would not have died" (John 11:21).

Can you hear the disappointment in her voice? Can you sense the rejection she must have felt? She must have thought He had hung up on her. But He didn't. He was still on the line even if He wasn't physically present. He was waiting to respond until Lazarus was dead so that God could be glorified in a greater way (John 11:4).

Your journey through grief may lead you through times when you wonder if God is still on the line. *God, where are You?* you ask. But all you hear is silence. Silence can make you feel uncomfortable. You may interpret it to mean that God has abandoned you. But has He really? Just because He hasn't responded in the way and timing you expected, does that mean He has hung up on you? Maybe He is waiting to respond in His timing and in His way.

You may not like that, but God has bigger plans. Perhaps God wants you to learn to trust Him through the silence. Does He want to reveal Himself to you in a different way?

Allow God to communicate to you through His silence. Learn to listen and wait. God says, "Never will I leave you; never will I forsake you" (Hebrews 13:5).

He is a God of truth. He never lies. He hasn't abandoned you or rejected you but is there even if you don't sense that He is. He is your Healer, and He wants to help you grow to know and trust Him more. Even if you don't hear from Him in the way you desire, He is there—listening, caring, feeling your pain.

Lord, where are You? You didn't respond in the way and timing I expected. I feel abandoned and hurt. I feel disconnected and distant from You. Are You listening? Silence makes me feel uncomfortable and rejected. Are You still on the line? Even though I can't see You, I know You are there. You say You will never leave me or forsake me. Please be my Healer. Help me to grow and trust You more. I want to know You through the silence. Show me how. Amen.

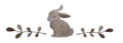

Steps Toward Healing

1. In what ways have you experienced God's silence in
   your grief journey? How has that made you feel?

_____

_____

_____

_____

_____

_____

2. Listen to His words. Read Psalm 4; Matthew 11:28–29;
   and Luke 6:20–49.

_____

_____

_____

_____

_____

_____

3. Read the story of Lazarus in John 11. Replace Martha's name with yours.

JESUS HAS A ROCKING CHAIR

I waited patiently for the LORD;
he turned to me and heard my cry.
He lifted me out of the slimy pit,
out of the mud and mire;
he set my feet on a rock
and gave me a firm place to stand.
He put a new song in my mouth.

PSALM 40:1–3

God, am I supposed to hurt this much?" I sobbed as I looked at the teddy bear sitting in my rocking chair. "I miss my baby."

Though often it seemed that God responded to my pleas with silence, that day God answered and encouraged me in an unexpected way. *It's probably another sympathy card,* I thought as I ripped open the envelope. Although I appreciated receiving cards and letters, that day was one of those times in my grief journey when I couldn't concentrate.

I felt relieved when I saw a hand-scribbled note from my cousin Crystal and a CD. Words through song had been Crystal's gift to others since her youth, when she and our troupe of cousins performed together. After several years our family ensemble dissolved, but Crystal and her sister, Debbie, continued music ministry together until Debbie died of cancer. Despite her pain and loss, Crystal chose to press on and continue singing. Her courage, perseverance, and ability to view her personal difficulties as the bass notes in her life's song had inspired me through the years.

Though distance has separated us for most of our lives, God has enabled Crystal and me to stay close in spirit, heart, and prayer. I sensed this CD was one more way God would intertwine our lives.

My curiosity mounted as I popped it in my player. Music filled the air, but I wasn't expecting what came next. I felt as if Crystal were sitting next to me, singing to my broken heart. Her words rang out, "He takes the place of Mom and Dad, He's the best parent a child could have. . . . Don't worry about the children, Jesus has a rocking chair. . . ."

As I pictured my child in the arms of Jesus, being rocked back and forth on the heavenly throne, peace filled my soul. Though I had never pondered a divine rocking chair before and had no evidence from Scripture that this was true, I did know that God was in control and could do anything, including using these timely lyrics to encourage me.

I sensed God's presence and compassion for me in a personal, powerful way that day. Each time I listen to Crystal's song, He continues to remind me that He loves and cares about every question I have about my loss. God is my Comforter and continues to use music to soothe my questioning soul.

Maybe it's time that you too allowed Him to comfort you through music. And while you're listening, picture yourself sitting on Jesus' lap. Feel His arms wrap tightly around you as you lay your head on His shoulder. Then He begins to rock . . . and rock . . . and rock.

Lord, am I supposed to hurt this much? My arms ache to hold and rock my child. I miss my precious baby. Will my life's song always be so sad? Meet me where I am today, and encourage me with Your truth. You are my song of hope. It's comforting to imagine that You could be holding my child in Your arms. Right now I need You to hold me. Wrap Your arms of peace around me, and rock away my fears. Put a new song in my heart. Amen.

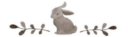

Steps Toward Healing

1. How do you feel when you picture Jesus in a rocking chair holding your child? Holding you?

_____

_____

_____

_____

_____

_____

2. What songs have soothed your soul during your grief journey?

_____

_____

_____

_____

3. God affirms music for your grieving soul. Consider the collection of songs and prayers in the book of Psalms. He inspired David and other writers to honestly pour out their hearts, questions, fears, and feelings. Find truth and comfort there. Read aloud Psalms 16, 17, and 23, or read the psalm that has encouraged you through your pain.

4. Listen to a song today. Select a praise song or a hymn, or download a popular song with encouraging lyrics. Listen. Then write down the lyrics and allow the words to soothe your soul.

_____

_____

_____

_____

Part 4

FORGIVING

Forgiving: *to pardon or acquit, to
cease to feel resentment against*

*When somebody you've wronged forgives you,
you're spared the dull and self-diminishing throb
of a guilty conscience. When you forgive somebody
who has wronged you, you're spared the dismal
corrosion of bitterness and wounded pride.*

FREDERICK BUECHNER

*Bear with each other and forgive one another
if any of you has a grievance against someone.
Forgive as the Lord forgave you.*

COLOSSIANS 3:13

Devotion 16

HIDDEN UNFORGIVENESS

Search me, God, and know my heart;
test me and know my anxious thoughts.
See if there is any offensive way in me,
and lead me in the way everlasting.

PSALM 139:23–24

*Y*our teeth look great. No cavities!"

I was surprised by my dentist's words. "Are you sure? Then why is my tooth so sensitive?" I asked. I knew *something* was wrong.

My dentist looked puzzled. He stared at my X-ray again. "Your tooth looks fine according to this. But let's take another look. Open wide."

I cringed when he placed the metal instrument on my tooth. *Tap. Tap. Tap.* "Ouch!" I exclaimed.

With a knowing look, my dentist motioned to his assistant. Moments later, my face was numb and the sound of a high-pitched drill filled the air. "I found the problem!" he said.

Hidden beneath my filling was a speck of decay. Although it was too small to detect on an X-ray, it was big enough to irritate the nerve in my tooth. I was relieved. The underlying cause of my pain was finally exposed and could be repaired before greater damage was done. I walked out of the dentist's office with a pain-free smile, renewed hope, and a new filling.

Your journey through grief may feel similar to a toothache at times. You may think you're coping with your loss fine until a person, place, thing, or event triggers a sensitive spot in you. *Ouch!* your heart says. Although you try to excuse your outbursts or rationalize your anger, the ache within your soul keeps getting worse. It may even keep you up at night.

When you ask others to diagnose your problem, they're shocked. They think you look great and appear to be handling your loss fine. Instinctively, however, you know *something* is wrong. So you decide to take a deeper look and ask God to help you.

What is causing my pain? you ask. You cringe when He

taps on your heart. Memories flood your mind. You recall the person who made thoughtless comments, the unfeeling doctor, the family member who ignored you, the friend who didn't call to tell you she is expecting, the spouse who wasn't sensitive to your pain.

With a knowing, loving look, the Lord softly replies, *Here's the problem—unforgiveness!* Hidden beneath my hurt is a part of me that doesn't want to forgive.

Although the resentments, anger, and disappointments I harbor against others seem small, if left undetected and untreated, the decay can destroy me. But if the underlying cause of my pain is finally exposed, with the Lord's help, it can be repaired. He holds out His nail-scarred hands and asks you to say as He said about His enemies, "Father, forgive them, for they do not know what they are doing" (Luke 23:34).

Have others wounded you with their words or actions? Is it possible that you are holding on to disappointment or resentment toward another person? Maybe it's time to explore what's hidden beneath your hurt. Is there a speck of unforgiveness there?

Invite the Lord to show you who you need to forgive. Get rid of the decay. Forgive. Ask Him to create a clean heart and renew a right spirit within you. Let Him replace your unforgiveness with His filling of love and forgiveness.

Then you can press on—relieved, restored, and ready to continue your healing journey.

God, I look as if I'm coping with my loss, but sometimes I overreact to people and circumstances. That's not like me. I know something is wrong. X-ray my heart and soul. Expose what's hidden there. Do I need to forgive someone? Show me who. Create a clean heart in me, and renew a right spirit within me. Fill me with Your love and forgiveness so I can continue my healing journey. Amen.

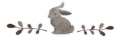

Steps Toward Healing

1. Have you been sensitive or overreacted to people or situations? If so, how? How is unforgiveness like decay if left untreated?

_____

_____

_____

_____

_____

_____

_____

2. Is there anyone you need to forgive? Who?

_____

_____

_____

_____

_____

_____

_____

3. God will enable you to forgive when you place
   your confidence in His ability. Read Isaiah 41:10 and
   Philippians 4:13. Say, "God, thank You for exposing my
   unforgiveness toward _____.
   I forgive _____ for

   _____

   _____

   _____."

Devotion 17

FORGIVING OTHERS

*"Father, forgive them, for they do not
know what they are doing."*

LUKE 23:34

Walt looked at his medical diploma hanging on his
office wall. *How many babies have I delivered in all
these years?* he wondered. He picked up a tiny bib on his
desk that said, "Dr. Walt saw me first." Faces of patients
flooded his mind . . . the first-time moms . . . the woman
who was forty-six and thought she had the flu . . . the
teenagers.

He recalled the poignant moments when he had to
share difficult news with some of his patients. "I'm sorry.

You've had a miscarriage." "Your tube has ruptured." "There is no heartbeat." "Your baby is going to die." A wave of compassion crashed in his heart as he recalled the look of disbelief in their eyes, the sorrow, the screams, the silence. Walt remembered how helpless he felt as he tried to comfort them. *Doctors are supposed to save lives, not lose them!* he thought. Although he knew that he had done everything humanly possible and that some things were out of his control, he still felt disappointed that he couldn't do more.

That's how he felt about Dottie. Just the mention of her name made his eyes fill with tears. She was one of those special patients who had touched his life deeply. *She was so excited when I told her she was pregnant with her first child,* he thought. *And when I told her a few weeks later that she had miscarried her child, I'll never forget how devastated she was.*

When Dottie discovered she was pregnant again, Walt was almost as excited as she was. But a few weeks later, that changed. His face grew solemn as he recalled the ultrasound report that revealed that Dottie's baby had a rare, fatal defect. He remembered how angry he felt because he couldn't fix her baby. And he was amazed when Dottie told him she would carry her child to term even though most in her situation would terminate the pregnancy.

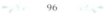

Walt talked honestly with Dottie about her forthcoming labor, delivery, and infant. He knew he couldn't fully prepare her to hold a dying baby. When Elizabeth was born, he was surprised at how Dottie, her friends, and her family lovingly celebrated the birth of this baby. "Dottie and Elizabeth" were the topic of discussion among most of the hospital staff during their brief stay. Walt was surprised at Dottie's inner strength and her insistence that she wanted to take her baby home. What amazed him even more was watching as more love lavished on Elizabeth during four days than most children receive in a lifetime. He couldn't quite put his finger on it, but he sensed that it had something to do with Dottie's God.

It wasn't until years later when Walt accepted God's forgiveness in his own life and was birthed into His kingdom that he realized what a significant role Dottie and Elizabeth had played in his journey to know God personally. Now Walt could understand the source of Dottie's inner strength. He knew that God was real and personal, the Great Physician who came to heal the spiritually sick and bind up the brokenhearted, the God who desires to save lives, who wants no one to perish.

God continued to transform Walt's heart. In time he realized that the disappointment, anger, and resentment he felt toward others needed to be released. *I need to forgive others even if I don't agree with their choices,* he thought. And he did, one patient at a time.

But he also prayed silently for his patients and was on call for God—ready to deliver a physical baby or a spiritual one.

I know because I was a recipient of Walt's prayers, support, and friendship when I walked the same path that my friend Dottie had trod years earlier. Ironically, I only knew him then as Dr. Walt, Dottie's doctor. But God chose to reconnect our lives through a friend when she announced her surprise engagement. I nearly fainted when I discovered that her husband-to-be was Dr. Walt. Only God could have orchestrated this.

I didn't know at the time how significant our friendship would become, but God did. He knew that Dr. Walt would become a vital support to our family and to my regular doctor during our journey through the valley of the shadow of death. God knew I would ask Dr. Walt to be my backup delivery doctor if my doctor was out of town when I went into labor. Even though Dr. Walt didn't deliver our child, somehow just knowing that he was willing to and would lovingly welcome our child into the world gave me peace.

Doctors and medical staff play a significant role in your loss experience. Maybe you've been wounded by their bedside manner, their insensitive comments, or their minimizing of your pain. Or did you have a caring doctor like Dr. Walt? If so, thank God for how He used your doctor.

Three years after the death of my son, my doctor finally shared with me an incident that still haunted him about my loss. "Kathe, do you remember when you had your baby and it was the change of shifts?" he asked.

I nodded.

"I'll never forget the thoughtless comment the new nurse made to you when you were holding your baby. She called your child an 'it' and 'abnormal.'" I could see the pain in his eyes.

By God's grace, I couldn't recall these words. But my doctor could. Three years later, it still hurt for him to talk about it.

"That's just like God, isn't it?" I said to my doctor. "To erase hurts from our hearts and memory." My doctor gave me a funny look as he nodded.

I'll never know fully how my words or actions through my journey of losing a child affected my doctor or others in the medical community. I can only hope that others saw a glimpse of the Great Physician through me and that my life reflected Jesus' words: "Father, forgive them, for they do not know what they are doing."

Are you holding anger or resentment toward your doctor, the medical staff, or others about your loss? Maybe there is just cause, or maybe they did everything they could for you and your baby. Only God knows. Maybe it's time to forgive those who have hurt you.

Who do you need to forgive? Allow the Great Physician to deliver you from your hurt and to help you release those from your grip of blame. Ask Him to birth a spirit of forgiveness in you and to reveal it to others.

God, You are the Great Physician. You ordain birth and death. Sometimes I expect too much from others. When I believe they let me down with their actions or comments, I feel anger and resentment toward them. Please show me the people I need to forgive who hurt me when I lost my child. Deliver me from my hurt, and help me release my blame. Birth a new spirit of forgiveness in me so I can truly say, "Father, forgive them, for they do not know what they are doing."

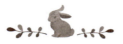

Steps Toward Healing

1. Do you blame anyone for your loss or for hurting you?

_____

_____

_____

_____

_____

_____

_____

2. List those you need to forgive.

_____

_____

_____

_____

_____

_____

_____

3. How do Jesus' words "Father, forgive them, for they do not know what they are doing" encourage you to do the same?

_____

_____

_____

_____

_____

_____

_____

4. Write Jesus' words in red letters over your list of names.

JOURNEY TO THE SNOWDRIFT OF FORGIVING YOURSELF

Set me free from my prison,
that I may praise your name.

PSALM 142:7

Kim rocked with grief. "Do something! Please do something. Help my baby!" she wailed. The doctors reassured her that there was nothing they could do to save her premature child. *This can't be happening*, she thought as she held her miniature son in her arms. *He looks perfect. He even has his daddy's face.* She counted his tiny fingers and toes. She stroked the hair on his apple-sized head.

She had longed for a son and had been the model patient

to maintain this pregnancy and stop the labor. She recalled her doctor's warning that if her baby was born too soon, he would not survive. She never dreamed she would have to face this circumstance. But as she watched her baby gasp for every breath and then lie still, she knew that her worst nightmare had come true. *My child is dead, and it's my fault!*

Like Kim, you may blame yourself for the loss of your child. *My body failed me and didn't fulfill its purpose. If only my hormone levels hadn't dropped. I didn't go to the hospital soon enough. I was too active and stressed. I made a wrong choice.*

You may feel as if you're "snowed in" by the winter storm of your grief. The icy winds of your memories blow against the door of your heart. The snow of self-blame keeps falling. Layer upon layer of guilt builds outside the door of your heart until the mound of your guilt is so high that you wonder if you'll ever be able to dig out. You're trapped. How will you get out?

In the book of Ruth, when Naomi lost her husband and two sons, I wonder if she felt snowed in by guilt and in some way responsible for their deaths. Did she heap layers of self-blame against the door of her heart? *If only I had refused to move here, they might still be alive. Because I condoned my sons marrying foreigners, God is punishing me.*

The wind of her sons' memories must have blown against the door of her heart every time she looked at her daughter-in-law Ruth. Ruth could have started a new life with the support of friends and family in her hometown in Moab. Instead, she traded certainty for an unknown future in a foreign land with an old woman.

Even the sound of her name, *Naomi*, which means "pleasant," made her cringe with guilt. "Call me Mara [Mara means bitter]," she said. "I went away full, but the LORD has brought me back empty" (Ruth 1:20–21).

Naomi's mound of guilt must have been so high outside the door of her heart that she didn't believe she would ever dig out, and it appeared as if she didn't want to. Was Naomi's guilt justified? Only God knows. How could she dig out of her snowdrift of guilt? She didn't know. But God did. He used her relative Boaz, a kinsman-redeemer, to help her.

I can only imagine how Naomi must have felt when Ruth came home after working in the fields and told Naomi about Boaz's acts of kindness. She must have been a bit reluctant to trust. Bitterness and self-blame felt more comfortable. Yet despite how she may have felt, Boaz continued to provide for Naomi and Ruth. Perhaps his love and faithfulness changed her heart and attitude, or maybe someone she knew confronted her. Did she hear a still, small voice whisper, *Naomi, it's time to free yourself from your past and your guilt and forgive yourself*?

I like to think God melted away Naomi's guilt and helped her see her need to trust Him and forgive herself. God replaced her blame with forgiveness and her mourning with joy.

God can do the same for you. Is a still, small voice calling your name? Listen. Can you hear Him saying, *It's time to free yourself from your guilt and forgive yourself*?

Your grief journey may lead you to a place where you need to forgive yourself. The concept of not letting go of anger, guilt, and condemnation toward yourself may be something you have never considered as sin that separates you from God. God will forgive you and will enable you to forgive yourself. Perhaps you even need to forgive yourself for needlessly placing blame on yourself.

Regardless of your circumstance, God understands. He is able to melt away the snow mound of guilt outside the door of your heart. He is your Kinsman-Redeemer, the One who offers you love, kindness, and forgiveness. Ask Him to dig through the snowdrift of your guilt and melt away the blame outside the door of your heart. He is ready to restore you so you can journey on.

Lord, I feel so guilty and often blame myself for losing my child. Although others try to comfort and console me, deep down I'm haunted by the thought that I could have done more or made different choices. I feel snowed in by my grief. The mound of my self-condemnation is so high outside the door of my heart that I feel as if I'll never be able to dig out. Help me, God. Enable me to forgive myself. Dig through the snowdrift of my guilt, and melt away my blame. You are my Kinsman-Redeemer, the One who has the power to set me free. Restore me today. Amen.

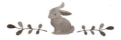

Steps Toward Healing

1. How do you feel guilty or blame yourself for the loss of your child?

_____

_____

_____

_____

_____

2. Have you forgiven yourself? If not, maybe it's time to share your feelings with God. Read 1 John 1:9.

_____

_____

_____

_____

_____

_____

_____

_____

_____

3. Now personalize 1 John 1:9: *I confess my sin of blaming myself for* _____. *God is faithful and just and has forgiven me for my sin and purified me from all unrighteousness. I am forgiven! Date* _____

4. Live forgiven. The next time you are tempted to blame yourself for the loss of your child, refer to this page.

Devotion 19

FORGIVING GOD

Why does this fellow talk like that? He's blaspheming!
Who can forgive sins but God alone?

MARK 2:7

Theresa was newly married and looking forward to starting a family. She dreamed of becoming a mother. When she discovered she was pregnant, she knew God had answered her prayer, so she threw a party to celebrate. She felt as if life couldn't get any better. But her fairy-tale life turned into a nightmare the day the pain in her side wouldn't subside and she was rushed to the hospital. She prayed that her baby would be safe.

When she woke up in the recovery room, her first question to her husband was, "Is our baby okay?"

He squeezed her hand as his eyes filled with tears. "Honey, I'm sorry. We couldn't save the baby. You had a tubal pregnancy. Surgery was necessary or we could have lost you."

At that moment Theresa wished that *she* was dead, not her baby. Over the next several months, her grief turned inward. Depression invaded her life. She avoided friends and family. Her appetite and sex drive diminished. Negative thinking and critical words became her new nature. Routine activities like climbing out of bed, dressing, and cooking exhausted her. She snapped at her husband for no apparent reason.

One day Theresa's friend Lynne ignored her excuses and showed up at her home anyway. "Get dressed!" Lynne announced. "We're going for a drive. It's time for you to come out of your cave of hibernation."

An hour later, Lynne and Theresa arrived at a lush parklike setting. Her friend got out of the car, opened her trunk, pulled out a red helium balloon, and handed it to Theresa. *What is this for?* Theresa thought as she followed Lynne to a nearby picnic table and sat down with her floating balloon. They talked for a while. Then Lynne leaned across the table, looked straight into Theresa's eyes, and asked, "Have you forgiven God?"

Theresa was stunned. She wasn't expecting *that* question.

"I've learned that there are usually three people we blame when life doesn't go according to our plans," Lynne said. "Ourselves . . . others . . . and God. From what you've told me, I don't believe you blame yourself, your husband, or the doctors for losing your child. So that only leaves God."

Theresa was silent. Somehow the thought of forgiving *God* felt wrong. She felt guilty for even entertaining the thought. But the more she pondered the idea of forgiving God, the more she wondered if her friend was right.

Lynne gave Theresa a knowing look as she handed her a thick black marker. "Theresa, take time to be alone with God right now and talk to Him. Tell Him what you're feeling, and ask Him to show you if you are angry at Him and need to forgive Him. Write a note to Him on your balloon with this marker and then release it," Lynne instructed. "And . . . don't worry, your balloon is environmentally safe!" she chuckled.

Theresa sat alone at the table. At first she felt uneasy talking to God because it had been a while. She listened and waited. Then she poured out her heart.

"God, You allowed my child to die. All I ever wanted was to be a mom!" she sobbed. She continued to share her hurts with Him until she had nothing more to say. Then she scribbled on her balloon, stood up, and released it. She watched the red ball ascend slowly, growing smaller with every passing minute until she could see only a speck in the sky, and then it was gone.

Theresa felt a soothing calm within her soul. She sensed that this was a healing moment in her grief journey. Finally she was at peace with God.

The concept of "forgiving God" can make many feel uneasy. It sounds prideful and self-righteous. Yet anger and bitterness toward God are far more common than most of us would like to admit. If we are honest about our anger toward God and admit the ways we feel He has let us down or has been unfair, then we can begin to heal.

Forgiving God doesn't mean He's guilty because He cannot commit any sin. But we need to destroy "every pretension that sets itself up against the knowledge of God, and . . . take captive every thought to make it obedient to Christ" (2 Corinthians 10:5).

Our thoughts may be rooted in perceptions of reality rather than in reality itself. When we forgive God, we release our expectations of what we *think* God should have done to prevent hurt, failure, or loss of any kind. God has big shoulders and allows us to vent. He wants us to tell Him how we feel so we can trust again. Satan is defeated when we stop pointing our finger at God and admit our false expectations.

Are you angry at God about your loss? Do you feel as if He let you down and should have intervened to change your situation? Even though God hasn't done anything wrong, do you feel as if you need to forgive Him? God understands. He suffered the loss of a child too.

Take time to talk to Him. Tell Him how you hurt. You too can grab a helium balloon and a marker if you want and write Him a note on the balloon, describing the ways you feel He let you down. Then release it. Go ahead. Let it go! Watch your unmet expectations float skyward until they disappear. Allow God's peace to soothe you as you continue to heal in your journey through grief.

God, I feel like You let me down. I'm hurt, disappointed, and angry at You for _____.
Please forgive me for thinking that I need to forgive You. You are sinless and perfect. Help me release to You my unmet expectations so that I can continue to heal. Amen.

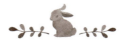

Steps Toward Healing

1. Forgiving yourself and others seems natural, but *forgiving God*? How does that concept make you feel?

_____

_____

_____

_____

_____

_____

2. Do you feel at times as if God let you down? In what ways? Tell Him.

_____

_____

_____

_____

_____

_____

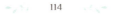

3. Take a thick marker and a helium balloon. Write on it the ways you feel God has let you down.

4. Ask God to help you release your balloon.

Devotion 20

RECEIVING THE
GIFT OF FORGIVENESS

*"For God so loved the world that he gave his
one and only Son, that whoever believes in
him shall not perish but have eternal life."*

JOHN 3:16

*G*ift giving is a fun Christmas tradition our family enjoys. As a child, I remember running to the
Christmas tree to search for packages that seemed to magi-
cally appear. I was elated one Christmas morning when I
discovered that the oversized box was for *me*. I can still
recall squealing with excitement when I looked inside and
realized the brown fluff of fur with the big red bow was a
puppy. At the time, I didn't fully comprehend or appreciate
how my gift was provided. However, I now realize that gift

giving has three essential elements: the Giver, the Gift, and the Receiver.

The Giver chooses and gives the gift. Motivated by an attitude of love or concern for the receiver, the giver's greatest desire is to know the receiver and give a meaningful, personal gift. That's what my parents did when they gave me a puppy. They selected a personal gift for me that they knew I had longed for.

The Gift comes at some cost or sacrifice to the giver and is free and unearned by those who receive it. My parents sacrificed time, money, trips to the vet, and sleep to give me a puppy.

The Receiver completes the gift-giving process when she accepts the gift into her possession. Only then does she receive the benefit of the giver's gift. I eagerly received my puppy with enthusiasm and joy!

Gifts, like puppies, come in all shapes and sizes. Most gifts are tangible, but some are not. Have you ever considered *forgiveness* as a gift? Pardoning or excusing others for wrongdoings and ceasing to feel resentment or anger toward them may be just what you need to do in your journey through grief.

Forgiveness may come wrapped in a variety of ways from different givers. One package may be from your spouse. It may come in the form of tears, an embrace, or an accepted apology after you hurled unkind words at him. Another package may contain a call, a card, or an invitation to have lunch from a friend or family member you ignored during the darkest days of your loss.

Tucked beneath the tree of your relationships may even be a package from the child you lost. *Do I need to seek forgiveness from my child?* you ask. Your child was a person too. If you feel you let your child down in some way, ask your child to forgive you. Although the contents of this package are void of actions or a response like the others, you can sense healing.

I admit that *giving* forgiveness is easier for me than receiving it. Maybe it's because *receiving* implies that *I* am guilty. *I am* the one who hurt or disappointed another person, and I need to make amends for the wrong I have done.

Some people may refuse to receive your gift of apology. If you have made every attempt to make amends, realize there may be nothing more you can do. You can't control how people respond, so don't try. Focus on what you can control. Take responsibility for your actions, your attitude, and your response to others. Leave the rest up to God. He can soften even the most hard-hearted person.

Although your gifts of forgiveness from others will be

packaged differently from mine, one shiny black gift with a big red bow marked "From God" is common to both of us and to every person who lives. God's motive in offering us this gift is pure, unconditional love for us. The gift He offers is free, unearned, and undeserved. It doesn't matter who you are, what you've done, or where you come from—God wants to give you this personal gift because He cares.

This shiny black package reminds us of how we "all have sinned and fall short of the glory of God" (Romans 3:23). Our sin and wrongdoings separate us from God. The big red bow reminds us that God's gift was made with great love and sacrifice: "For God so loved the world that he gave his one and only Son, that whoever believes in him shall not perish but have eternal life" (John 3:16). Jesus died on the cross for your sins and mine, and He rose again so that we can live with God forever.

Have you received God's gift of eternal life and His forgiveness by believing in Jesus? If so, thank Him for this gift. If not, maybe it's time. God wants you to have this gift. He loves you so much. Go ahead. Accept it.

When you do, lift the lid off the box and look inside. It's white and empty. That's the way God sees you now—clean, without sin, forgiven. He will help you keep it that way—one situation and one person at a time.

Why not start right now? Ask Him to help you see who you have wronged, and then ask for forgiveness. Forgiveness is a gift for you to receive from God and from others—and to give as well. Why not pass it on to someone else?

God, thank You for reminding me that giving and receiving forgiveness is a necessary part of my healing journey. Tucked beneath the tree of my relationships are people I have hurt. From whom do I need to receive the gift of forgiveness? Please forgive me for how my thoughts, words, and actions have wounded others. My expectations and conditional love got in the way. Give me courage to tell others I'm sorry and ask them to forgive me. Remind me each time I look at a wrapped gift that You gave me an oversized gift I didn't deserve—Your life. Thank You for wrapping Yourself around my sins and for willingly dying on a cross for me. Your bow of sacrifice demonstrates Your unconditional love for me. I accept Your gift. Give me courage to admit my wrongs to others and to receive their gift of forgiveness too. Amen.

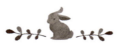

Steps Toward Healing

1. What was your favorite Christmas gift as a child? How did you feel when you opened it?

_____

_____

_____

_____

_____

_____

2. Do you most enjoy giving gifts or receiving them? Why?

_____

_____

_____

_____

_____

_____

3. Is it easier for you to give forgiveness or receive it? Why?

_____

_____

_____

_____

_____

_____

_____

4. Think about God's gift of forgiveness wrapped up under the tree of eternal life. The tag has your name on it.

To: _____ *From: God*

What draws you to open it? What makes you reluctant to accept it?

_____

_____

_____

_____

_____

_____

RECEIVING THE GIFT OF FORGIVENESS

5. Who have you hurt with your words, thoughts, or actions, and from whom do you need to ask for the gift of forgiveness?

To: _____

From: _____

Tell them. Give them the gift of "I'm sorry. Will you please forgive me?" and receive the gift from them.

Part 5

RELATING

Relating: *to tell, show, establish a logical or casual association, connect with*

Praise be to the God and Father of our Lord Jesus Christ, the Father of compassion and the God of all comfort, who comforts us in all our troubles, so that we can comfort those in any trouble with the comfort we ourselves receive from God.

2 CORINTHIANS 1:3–4

We go through what we go through to help others go through what we went through.
KATHE WUNNENBERG, *Hopelifter: Creative Ways to Spread Hope When Life Hurts*

Devotion 21

WHO DO YOU SAY THAT I AM?

[Jesus] asked his disciples. . . . "Who do you say I am?" Simon Peter answered, "You are the Messiah, the Son of the living God."

MATTHEW 16:13, 16

"ow many children do you have?" the waiter asked as he handed me the menu.

His question startled me. But before I could say a word, however, my son Jake said with confidence, "Seven! Four in heaven and three on earth!" I don't know who was more surprised—me, my husband, or the waiter.

As you journey through grief, you may find yourself in unexpected situations where you need to communicate your loss with others. Like ordering from a menu at a restaurant, you have a multitude of options from which to choose. The depth of your sharing about your loss is up to you. You may choose to share little, much, or not at all. Your decision may depend on the circumstances or on the people involved in each encounter.

When Jesus asked His disciples, "Who do people say the Son of Man is?" I wonder if they felt caught off guard and awkward. How should they respond to Jesus? Their responses were varied.

"Some say John the Baptist; others say Elijah; and still others, Jeremiah or one of the prophets."

Jesus went on to ask them, "But what about you? Who do you say that I am?"

Simon Peter replied, "You are the Messiah, the Son of the living God."

I can sense the confidence in the way Peter proclaimed his answer. He spoke without hesitation. Did Peter anticipate being asked this question? Had he predetermined what he would say? Although the Bible doesn't tell us, I think it's safe to assume that Peter was comfortable with his response and spoke honestly. He shared the truth.

I have discovered that it is helpful to anticipate the situations in which you may be asked pointed questions and to plan your response. What will you say? How much will you share? With whom will you share? How will you refer to your child? How will you refer to yourself? Do you know what your husband or children will say about your loss?

Advance planning can prevent hurt feelings or awkward moments. Feeling comfortable with words that describe your child or loss experience can help you relate your loss to others in a positive and healthy way. Communication can be a healing part of your journey through grief.

Who do you say that you are since you've lost a child? Are you still a mother even though you have empty arms? Are you a mother of one, two, three, or more?

Who do you say your child is? Your son or daughter? A gift from God? That's a question only you can answer and relay to others.

And who do you say Jesus is? How you respond to this question has eternal consequences. I hope that you, like Peter, say with confidence, "You are the Messiah, the Son of the living God, my Lord and Savior."

God, how should I communicate my loss to others? Sometimes I feel uncomfortable and tongue-tied. I want to speak with ease. Please show me how. Guide my words with Your wisdom. Prepare me to respond to others. Who do You say that I am? Thank You for being my Father and for sending Your Son, Jesus, to die for me. I can say with confidence that I will spend eternity with You as Your child. Amen.

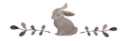

Steps Toward Healing

1. How has loss changed you?

_____

_____

_____

_____

_____

2. What new insights has God shown you about yourself?

_____

_____

_____

_____

_____

3. Who do you say that you are? How can you
   express that to others?

_____

_____

_____

_____

_____

4. You will always be a child of God, regardless of the
   changes in your life. How does that make you feel?
   How does your experience of loss give you new
   opportunities to share your identity in Him with others?

_____

_____

_____

_____

_____

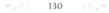

Devotion 22

HE'LL MEET YOU
WHERE YOU ARE

*"Are not two sparrows sold for a penny?
Yet not one of them will fall to the
ground outside your Father's care. And
even the very hairs of your head are all
numbered. So don't be afraid; you are
worth more than many sparrows."*

MATTHEW 10:29–31

"KATH, COME QUICK!"

I knew by the tone of my husband's voice that something was terribly wrong as I waddled through the backyard toward him and Jake, our six-year-old son.

"It's a baby bird!" sobbed Jake as he knelt on the ground.

I stepped closer, and then I saw the spoon-sized, featherless creature lying next to a clump of twigs.

My husband's eyes dimmed with disappointment. "I had no idea a baby bird was in the nest!"

Jake looked up at me. Tears streamed down his face. "Mom, can we save him?"

How I longed to tell my son in that moment what he desired to hear—that I could miraculously heal this baby bird—but I could not. As traumatic as this moment was, I knew I must tell him the truth. "No, Jake. I'm sorry. The baby bird is dead," I solemnly replied. Then I knelt down, wrapped my arms around my son, and cried with him.

The baby bird was Jake's first personal encounter with death. I couldn't minimize this experience or the pain he was feeling, so I met him where he was and joined him in his grief encounter. Together our family buried the baby bird and thanked God for its brief life. Ironically, three weeks later, we stood together once again, but this time at a cemetery, where we thanked God for the brief life of our child.

Was this a coincidence, or was this God's way of meeting us where we were? I'll never know for sure in this lifetime, but I do know that Jesus is a relational expert. He touches people where they are and communicates to them in unique ways they can understand. He met the woman at the well at midday because He knew that's when a woman with her reputation would be there. James and John were working by the seashore when Jesus met them and invited them to become "fishers of men." He hung between two criminals, one of whom accepted His offer to join Him in Paradise.

Encounters with Jesus were often simple, ordinary moments, like when He shared about a farmer sowing seeds, about sheep and about goats, and about a vine and its branches. His actions and words met listeners where they were and related truth in a way they could understand and apply.

His words still do that. Maybe that's why God chose to use a baby bird to relate death to Jake and prepare him for losing his baby brother. God met him where he was and communicated truth to him in a powerful, meaningful way.

How we choose to relate our loss to others is personal and unique for each of us. I've discovered that honest communication works best in our family. We give one another permission to be where we are in our grief journey, which may mean handing a tissue to the one in tears or having a picnic on a grave. It may mean enduring silence or words, anger or laughter.

Sometimes we choose to celebrate and honor the children we have lost through special ornaments on our Christmas tree, scholarships for needy children, anonymous gifts to families in crisis, sharing our story with others, or giving yellow rubber ducks as baby gifts to others. Though others aren't usually aware of the significance of the duck they've received, I am. It reminds me of the baby bird God used to touch our hearts and help prepare us for the loss of our child. It prompts me to thank God for relating to me in a personal, meaningful way and encourages me to do the same with others. God continues to meet me where I am. He will do the same for you.

Precious Lord, thank You for demonstrating Your love for me in specific ways and for being my Companion through my hiding, suffering, and questioning. You are the One who knows when every bird falls to the ground. You know the number of hairs on my head. You care about me personally and meet me where I am. Continue to guide me and be my Companion as I journey through relating to others. Amen.

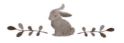

Steps Toward Healing

1. What specific situation or person has God used to meet you in your grief? What did you learn? Why was this encounter meaningful?

_____

_____

_____

_____

_____

2. Think about the people Jesus encountered in the books of Matthew, Mark, Luke, and John. Which person or story can you relate to? Why?

_____

_____

_____

_____

_____

3. If you could honor or celebrate the child you never knew, what would you do? How could you include your circle of family or friends?

_____

_____

_____

_____

_____

Devotion 23

JOURNEY THROUGH THE SEASONS OF FRIENDSHIP

That person is like a tree planted by streams of water, which yields its fruit in season.

PSALM 1:3

I love trees! They refresh me and soothe my soul. They provide shade from the heat, shelter from the rain, and a place to hide, climb, or build a tree house. When transition is thrust on them through the seasons, they adapt. Trees mature in summer and change colors and drop leaves in fall. They know when to shut down to survive winter and when to sprout new beginnings in springtime. Some trees, like the sequoias in northern California, grow in clusters. Their roots web together, enabling them to withstand strong, blustery winds.

Like trees, you will need to endure different seasons in your grief. There will be times when you will need to be rooted in a support system of relationships.

Often through the years and in my grief journey I have felt guilty and uncaring about not maintaining friendships the way I thought I should. My list of expectations included remembering birthdays, meeting regularly, sharing meaningful conversation, and writing or calling often.

I was freed from this slavery of expectations when I heard a friend share about the seasons of friendship. She told me that it is normal to have different friendships through different seasons in one's life. Some are with you through childhood, singleness, and college. Others come alongside when you start your career, marriage, or family. Some friends spend a season with you to help you grow spiritually or to support you through a change or crisis. And some are friends with you through your grief, whether in presence or in memory.

That's how God used Dottie in my life—as a friend who modeled how to grieve the loss of a child. Several years ago, I walked through Dottie's miscarriage and her baby's death with her. Throughout the months of her pregnancy with a baby with a fatal birth defect, I observed her live her faith. She welcomed me into her intimate journey of the birth and death of her daughter, Elizabeth, and allowed me to experience her journey through grief. A move separated us and we lost touch as friends. Years later, when I discovered that my baby would die with the same birth defect as Dottie's, I knew I could make it through because she had. God used her friendship from a past season to comfort me and give me courage.

Jesus wants us to make the most of our seasons of friendship. He met people in the season of life when they needed Him most. Picture the paralytic, the leper, the blind man. The twelve disciples needed Jesus' friendship to teach them, and Jesus knew they would need one another's as well.

Jesus is your caring, faithful Friend during this season of your life when you need Him most. He will never leave you or forsake you, and He will be your Friend for all seasons. He has provided others to support you during this time in your life. He may also bring to mind friends from seasons past, like my friend Dottie was to me, who can encourage you now. Your Jesus-with-skin-on friends will walk with you through your pain and are tangible reminders of His love and concern for you. In time, you'll be able to support others who need a friend for a time or season. Stay close to Jesus. He will guide you.

God, thank You for the gift of my friends and for the seasons of friendship with them. Sometimes You place a person in the springtime of my life when I need a new perspective. Or You use friends to help me grow and mature. When I need to change or let go, my autumn friends are there for me. And some friends allow me to shut down and be still in the winter of my grieving. They know when to release the friendship. Thank You for the friends past, present, and future whom You provide. Thank You for drawing close to me in every season of my grieving. Direct me to those who need a friend for a season in their grief. Use me to encourage them. Amen.

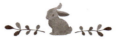

Steps Toward Healing

1. If you don't have friends for this season of grief, ask God to connect you to someone or remind you of a person from your past whose example could encourage you (it could be someone from the Bible).

_____

_____

_____

_____

2. Who are the friends who understand your personal experience and grief and are with you in the journey? Which friends:

• Give you new perspectives?

_____

_____

_____

_____

• Help you grow and mature?

_____

_____

_____

_____

_____

_____

• Support you through change?

_____

_____

_____

_____

_____

_____

• Encourage you to slow down and be still?

_____

_____

_____

_____

_____

3. Who can you be a friend to through her season
   of grieving? Ask God to show you someone you can
   invest in for a season.

_____

_____

_____

_____

_____

4. God is a Friend for all seasons. How do you most
   need Him to help you this week? To give you new
   perspectives? To help you grow and mature? To
   support you through change? To encourage you to
   slow down and be still?

_____

_____

_____

_____

_____

PLAYMATES IN HEAVEN

"Love one another. As I have loved you,
so you must love one another."

JOHN 13:34

*G*od often will bring people across your path who can relate to your loss.

I couldn't have known that God would answer my prayers to fill the house next door with a friend who understood my broken heart. Just weeks after our baby's death, we saw a family walk out of the house next door. *Could these be our new neighbors?* I wondered. We smiled and waved. They smiled and waved back. "Are you interested in the house?" we asked.

They nodded and walked closer. We told them that the best part of buying the house would be having us as neighbors! We all laughed. Then I noticed their two-year-old daughter and a small white bundle in the woman's arms. "How old is your baby?" I asked.

"Three months," she replied.

What a coincidence, I thought. *Our baby would be two months old.*

A few days later we saw the Sold sign. The young family we met would indeed be our new neighbors. Stephanie, the mother, was just the person I needed for this season of my life. She had experienced the death of an infant son a year earlier. His name was Jacob, our living son's name.

God knew exactly what He was doing by connecting our lives. How comforting to have a friend next door who understood my joy, my sorrow, and my journey through grief. For several years, while we were neighbors, on my son John Samuel's birthday I could count on a card, a hug, or a gift from Stephanie. It meant so much to know *someone* remembered. Two days later, on her son Jacob's birthday, I would reciprocate.

One year I suggested we go to a lake to commemorate Jacob's life. We sang "Happy Birthday," and then she and her children released balloons and threw flowers in the lake. As her children frolicked by the water, I sat across from Stephanie at a picnic table and listened to her pour out her mother heart. I understood her sorrow and her joy.

"Maybe our boys are playmates in heaven!" I said.

We both smiled at the thought of our sons running through the streets of gold, hearing stories about the Flood from Noah himself, and sitting side by side with Jesus.

Even though we can't know for sure that this is true, it's a comforting thought. What I do know is that God is sovereign and is the divine Connector. He intertwined my life with Stephanie's at a time in my grief journey when I needed someone to relate to and understand my mother-heart.

Connecting with others who understand your loss can provide healing. You may receive encouragement or you may give it. Do you know someone who has also lost a child? If not, ask God to connect you to someone. He wants us to encourage one another in our journey through grief. Maybe your child and mine are playmates in heaven. Only God knows. But one day, we too will know for sure.

God, You are the divine Connector. You have a purpose and a plan for the people You have placed in my life. Thank You for caring about me and for others who care too. Help me be sensitive to others who have lost a child and encourage them. Lead me to those You want me to meet. Amen.

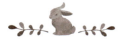

Steps Toward Healing

1. Read 2 Corinthians 3–4; Galatians 6:2; Ephesians 4:32; and 1 Thessalonians 4:18.

_____

_____

_____

_____

_____

_____

_____

_____

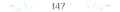

2. How does God want you to respond to others who are grieving?

_____

_____

_____

_____

_____

3. Who has lost a child and would appreciate your encouragement? How will you do this?

_____

_____

_____

_____

_____

Due dates, birthdays, anniversaries, holidays, Mother's Day, and Father's Day can be painful days for those who have lost a child. Consider ways you can show comfort to others on those occasions. For unique ideas, check out my recipes of hope from my book *Hopelifter: Creative Ways to Spread Hope When Life Hurts*, or go to www.hopelifters.com.

Devotion 25

IT'S PITCHER-FILLING TIME!

*May the God of hope fill you with all joy and peace
as you trust in him, so that you may overflow
with hope by the power of the Holy Spirit.*

ROMANS 15:13

The experience of loss can drain the energy from your life and leave you feeling so empty that you are unable to relate to others in a positive way. *I have nothing left to give,* you think. And in most cases, you're probably right.

I've experienced seasons like this. Meeting the needs of others comes naturally for me, so when I was unable to do this with joy on one specific occasion, I knew I needed help. I went through my checklist:

☐ Am I eating properly?

☐ Am I getting enough rest?

☐ Are hormones an issue?

☐ Do I have too much activity in my life?

☐ Is exercise a part of my regular routine?

☐ Do I have hidden hurt? (I even explored the possibility of unforgiveness, anger, guilt, or resentment toward others who may have caused me pain and who I need to forgive.)

☐ Is a trigger date, holiday, or significant event approaching? (Often I feel drained around the anniversary dates when I lost my children or at times when I should be experiencing their significant milestones, like learning to crawl, or walk, starting school, playing sports, or graduating.)

I sought medical attention, and my physical examination resulted in a healthy, normal report.

Ironically, it was my friend Patty who helped me solve my problem when I was attending her workshop. Patty picked up a pitcher filled with water and began to pour it into several glasses. She compared this to how we pour out our lives to other people each day: our families, job, friends in crisis, and activities. Sooner or later we become dry. *This is exactly how I feel!* I thought.

Then Patty asked, "What are you doing to *fill* your pitcher so you can continue to pour out into others?"

Fill my pitcher? I had never considered that before. After all, I'm a doer. I like to encourage others, but taking time to fill *my* emotional pitcher with people, places, or things that energize *me* seemed selfish. Was Patty right?

Since I'm the type of person who has to learn through experience, I decided to try what she suggested. I went home and made a list of "pitcher-filling" items:

- reading a book
- talking with a friend
- getting away for a weekend to enjoy pine trees and snow
- receiving a manicure and pedicure
- having the night off as Mom
- dining out with my husband
- drinking a frothy cappuccino
- enjoying uninterrupted time alone with God

Then I determined that I would fill my pitcher the next week and be intentional about doing a few things

Grieving the *Child* I Never Knew

that energized me. By the end of the week I was amazed at how much better I felt. I was able to laugh again and serve others with a smile. Others noticed my change too and wondered what had happened. "I filled my pitcher!" I answered.

Self-care is important in your journey through grief. Although losing a child may be a onetime event, your loss will have a ripple effect that can last a lifetime. Just when you think you're doing great, a situation or person may trigger a painful memory of losing your child and you feel as if your emotional pitcher is being drained. Because I continued to struggle with self-care and desired to make it a priority, I finally sought professional help and hired a life coach to meet with on the phone most weeks (I still do this!).

Be gentle with yourself through the process. If you feel drained of energy and can't find a reason why, is it possible that you've been pouring out so much for others that your emotional pitcher is empty and needs to be filled? Have you neglected spending time with God and allowing Him to fill your spiritual pitcher?

God wants you to live life to the full so that you can serve others cheerfully. But He also wants you to love yourself as much as you love others and to take time for self-care. Even Jesus knew when to stop in order to fill His pitcher. He took time to play, laugh, fish, sleep, and spend time alone with God. He kept pouring out His life for others, but He was able to do that because He knew when and how to keep His pitcher full.

What about you? Have you been pouring into others so much that you've neglected yourself? Has your loss required you to pour out emotionally even more? Are you drained spiritually and need to be filled? Maybe it's time to fill *your* pitcher. Do something this week that will energize you. Spend time with God, and ask Him to fill you spiritually and reveal to you people, places, or things that may encourage you. He wants you to live life energized and to the full. Ask Him to show you how.

God, I'm drained. I feel as if my pitcher is dry and I have nothing left to give to others. Help me love myself and take time for self-care. Show me specific ways that I can fill my pitcher. Draw me close to You and fill me spiritually. It's pitcher-filling time, Lord. Fill me up with Your love so I can pour it out to others. Amen.

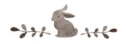

Steps Toward Healing

1. How are you pouring out to others daily?

_____

_____

_____

_____

2. God tells us to love our neighbors as ourselves. How
   are you demonstrating self-care?

_____

_____

_____

_____

3. How do you know if your pitcher is empty?

_____

_____

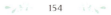

_____

_____

_____

4. Make a list of specific ways that you or others
   can nourish or energize you.

_____

_____

_____

_____

_____

Part 6

SEEKING

Seeking: *to search for, request, aim, or try*

> *"Ask and it will be given to you; seek
> and you will find; knock and the
> door will be opened to you."*

MATTHEW 7:7

Seek God in your darkness, and He will be your light.
Seek God in your questions, and He will be your answer.
Seek God in your anger, and He will be your peace.
Seek God in your sorrow, and He will be your comforter.
Seek God in your uncertainty, and He will be your confidence.
Seek God in your sin, and He will be your redeemer.
Seek God in your forgiveness, and He will be your salvation.
Seek God in your salvation, and He will be your eternity.

KATHE WUNNENBERG

Devotion 26

SEEING BEYOND
YOUR CLOUD OF LOSS

"For I know the plans I have for you,"
declares the LORD, "plans to prosper you
and not to harm you, plans to give you
hope and a future. Then you will call on
me and come and pray to me, and I will
listen to you. You will seek me and find me
when you seek me with all your heart. I
will be found by you," declares the LORD.

JEREMIAH 29:11–14

*L*ook up! What do you see?" I asked as I pointed to the
puffs of white landscaped across the turquoise sky.
"An elephant! A submarine!" squealed my son Jake.
"Mom, look at that whale! Dad, what do *you* see?"

158

Silence pervaded the car. I sensed that my engineer-minded husband was not in the mood to play "name that cloud" for the next hundred miles of our trip.

Jake persisted. "Come on, Dad . . ."

Finally, Rich responded, "I don't see anything—but clouds!"

Clouds fascinate me. Unlike my husband, I love to watch them transform and to imagine what they might become. When I look up, I see beyond a mass of water or ice particles that appears as floating mist or fog to a theater in the sky. The blue backdrop sets the stage for the clouds of changing cast and props.

How we view our loss is a lot like looking at clouds. We may see only the floating fog of sorrow, or we can choose to look beyond it to a future in the process of being shaped. Eventually we reach a point in our grief journey when we must decide whether we will allow God to transform our lives through loss. He knows the plans He has for us, to give us hope and a future. He knows what He will show us. But first we must look up and trust God wholeheartedly with our uncertainty.

I remember the day I made that decision. Our family and friends had gathered to praise God for the brief life of our son. As I stared at the teddy bear with three helium balloons

GRIEVING THE *Child* I NEVER KNEW

sitting on the altar, I thought about my child and the plans and future I would never experience with him in this lifetime. I would never see him take his first step, crash on his bike, play catch with his brother, drive his first car, graduate from high school, marry, or have a child of his own. My plans to read books to him, sing lullabies, and teach him to pray would never come to pass. Would I allow this cloud of loss to cast a shadow on the rest of my life? I knew that was a decision only I could make. *But how do I see beyond it?* I wondered.

We gave helium balloons to our guests to release as they left. I decided to cling to mine as I walked outside. Then I looked up. Clouds were everywhere. *They're beautiful!* I thought. At that moment I sensed God telling me to let go of my loss, so I released my balloon. As I watched it ascend toward the clouds, I felt my spirit lifting and hope returning to me. I knew that God had plans for my future and would help me see beyond my cloud of loss. I did not know at the time that He would transform my loss into books, speaking, and a Hopelifters ministry to mentor others, but He did.

When Christ died, the cloud of loss must have overshadowed the disciples. Did they feel as if their hopes, plans, and futures had been erased? Would they ever see beyond the tomb? I can hardly imagine the hurt and hopelessness they must have felt. Disappointment must have dimmed their view.

But three days later, Christ rose from the grave. He defeated death. He transformed their cloud of loss into a future with hope. Did their spirits soar as they looked up and watched Jesus ascend into the clouds to join His Father in heaven?

Someday when we least expect it, Jesus will come back. I wonder how it will feel on that day to look up at the theater in the sky and see Jesus, center stage, riding on His chariot of clouds.

Maybe it's time for you to look up and invite Him to help you see beyond your loss. He is the Alpha and Omega, the One who is, who was, and who is to come. He knows the plans He has for you, to give you hope beyond your hurt and a future not bound by your past. Why not ask Him today? Release your cloud of loss to Him, and watch Him begin to transform your life.

God, thank You for clouds. They remind me that You are in the process of shaping my future. Help me trust You wholeheartedly and see beyond my loss to the plans You have for me. Transform my hurt into healing, my fear into faith, and my past into a future with hope. I release it to You today. You are the Alpha and Omega, the One who is, who was, and who is to come. Remind me to look up as we journey on. Amen.

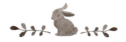

Steps Toward Healing

1. Jesus is the One who transforms lives. In what area(s) of your life (physically, emotionally, socially, or spiritually) has He transformed you the most through your loss?

_____

_____

_____

_____

_____

_____

2. In what area do you still need to seek His hope?

_____

_____

_____

_____

_____

_____

SEEING BEYOND YOUR CLOUD OF LOSS

3. What plans do you sense God may have for you
   in the future?

   _____

   _____

   _____

   _____

   _____

4. Read the verse at the beginning of this devotion
   and rewrite it here, inserting your name.

   _____

   _____

   _____

   _____

   _____

   _____

   _____

   _____

   _____

   _____

   _____

Devotion 27

DO YOU WANT TO GET WELL?

He heals the brokenhearted and
binds up their wounds.

PSALM 147:3

First one in gets healed!" could have been the motto of the people at the pool of Bethesda. The area was landscaped with many blind, lame, and paralyzed people, each hoping to be restored by the healing waters. The stench of unclean bodies and salve filled the air. Most were beggars lying in the rut of despair with no desire or hope for a better future.

One invalid had been there for thirty-eight years. His problem had apparently become a way of life for him. No one had ever helped him, and he had lost hope of ever being healed. Jesus approached him and asked, "Do you want to get well?" (John 5:6).

You'd think the man would have shouted, "Yes!" Instead, he responded with excuses. Maybe he was afraid of being healed. Healing would mean a new way of life for him. No more begging. How would he get food? He would have to take care of himself and go to work. Did he feel anxious about change and prefer living in the comfort zone of hopelessness?

"Then Jesus said to him, 'Get up! Pick up your mat and walk.' At once the man was cured; he picked up his mat and walked" (vv. 8–9).

You may feel as if your grief has paralyzed you emotionally or spiritually. No matter how trapped you feel in your infirmities from your loss, God can minister to your deepest needs. Don't let your loss cause you to lose hope for the future. God may have special work for you to do—in spite of your loss or because of it.

- Helen Keller allowed others to see God through her blindness.
- God uses Joni Eareckson Tada's paralysis to help others walk spiritually.

- After her premature twins, Arie and Hadilyn, died, Shayla started a box ministry that provides families in the hospital with practical, meaningful items to comfort them as they prepare to say good-bye to their baby.
- God used Kim and Debbie to start and lead support groups in their church, using this book to encourage grieving moms, bringing purpose to the pain of the losses of Kim's daughter, Narissa, and Debbie's son, Shaun. Kim also mentors others who desire to start a group.
- Gia and her family started a foundation to encourage grieving families after Sable died. Funding and furnishing a comfort room in a hospital for bereaved families and sponsoring Hopelifters annual bus trips for mothers who have lost children are examples of some of their support.
- Gloria reached out to encourage the nurses who cared for her and her son, Peter, by giving them personalized gifts. She also began sharing her story with individuals and groups.
- Heather started running to manage her grief after losing baby Bowen to polycystic kidney disease. She runs marathons and raises money for this cause and supports children on dialysis in practical ways.

- Karen and Becky started an annual conference for women who long for or have lost a child. Both became certified Christian doulas to help others walk through the paralysis of preparing to lose a child.

Do you want to get well? This is a question you have to ask yourself. Do you want Jesus to heal the areas in your life where you have been wounded by your loss? Or do you want to keep hiding, suffering, questioning, and blaming? Are you comfortable living with your anger, hurt, or depression, or are you ready to seek restoration for your future?

You may be holding tightly to the things that are paralyzing you spiritually. Is it time to forgive yourself or others? Do you need to invite Jesus to come near? Christ can heal all the areas of your life. But if He does, you'll need to let go of your excuses.

Jesus doesn't accept your excuses or see you as you see yourself—lying in a rut of despair. He sees your potential. Through His grace, He will work through your loss in the future. He is reaching out His hand to you. "Do you want to get well?" He asks. "Get up and walk."

Go ahead. Seek His healing. Get up and walk. Embrace your future. Allow God to transform your hurt into hope for others.

Lord, I've been paralyzed in my grief and am lying in a rut of despair. I'm tired of hiding, suffering, questioning, and blaming. I need Your healing. Please forgive me for resisting Your touch. I want to get well! Replace my sorrow with joy, my anger with peace, my hopelessness with hope, and my pain with purpose. Help me get up and walk into the future and, in Your perfect plan and timing, help others. Amen.

Steps Toward Healing

1. Read the story in John 5. Imagine you are the person Jesus approached and asked, "Do you want to get well?" How will you respond to Him?

_____

_____

_____

_____

_____

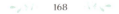

2. What excuses have paralyzed you from fully healing and moving forward?

_____

_____

_____

_____

_____

3. Maybe now is the time to get up and walk into your future! What steps can you take to start?

_____

_____

_____

_____

_____

4. Invite God to transform your hurt into hope to help others. What ideas come to mind?

_____

_____

_____

_____

Devotion 28

HOLDING HANDS
WITH YOUR FUTURE

"So do not fear, for I am with you;
do not be dismayed, for I am your God.
I will strengthen you and help you;
I will uphold you with my
righteous right hand."

ISAIAH 41:10

When Mark and Karen discovered she was expecting triplets, they were surprised and delighted but also apprehensive. They knew how risky this type of pregnancy could be.

Nineteen weeks into the pregnancy, Karen's water broke and she was rushed to the hospital. Their tiny son, Morgan, was born and, within a few hours, died.

"You can expect to lose the other two within forty-eight hours," the doctor announced.

Mark and Karen felt as if they were slipping into a hole of hopelessness. Could they climb out of it only to face the future with more loss? Family and friends from coast to coast sought God through prayer. Prayer was the lifeline of hope that pulled them out of their despair. Miraculously, Karen's contractions stopped, and she began to feel more hopeful that her two remaining babies would be saved. "Don't be too optimistic," the doctor told the couple. "Only a handful of children throughout the world have ever survived a situation like yours."

"The doctors are looking only at the medical side," Mark whispered to Karen. "They aren't putting God into the equation."

Over the next several days, Karen underwent several medical procedures and finally was sent home on bed rest. Although the doctors thought Mark and Karen were not grasping reality, the couple felt as if God was holding them tightly in the grip of His grace. Friends and family rallied to support them with meals, lawn care, cards, and letters.

Karen felt relieved when week twenty-five finally arrived. *My babies can almost survive,* she thought. She wondered what it would feel like in the future when she was able to sit and hold them on the sofa instead of lie on it. *Just a few more weeks . . .*

But Karen's labor started again, and a week later her doctor performed an emergency C-section. Laura and Sarah were born, each weighing one pound, twelve ounces. Though severely premature, both girls responded well to early treatments. Each day that passed was one day closer to a hopeful future. When the babies reached the two-week milestone, Karen and Mark knew their chances of survival were excellent.

But late one night a nurse called. "Laura is sick. Come immediately!"

Mark and Karen found themselves back on the merry-go-round of emotions, holding tightly to the uncertainty about their future. Would this ride ever stop? During the next several hours, Mark and Karen watched and prayed. They felt so helpless. Sitting at the hospital and watching his daughter fight for her life was not how Mark imagined spending his first Father's Day. But as he sat there, he was filled with compassion as his daughter looked up at him and grasped his finger with her tiny hand.

"You know how to get to your daddy's heart!" he said.

During the course of Laura's time in the hospital, Mark recalled the many times she had given him "that look" with her eyes as if she wanted to hold hands. So Mark would extend his finger, and she would grasp it. They held hands as long as Laura wanted to. Sometimes holding hands with his daughter meant being late for work, but Mark didn't mind. "Someday I'll teach you to ride a bike and fish. Hang in there, little girl," he whispered.

Several transfusions and hours later, the doctor announced, "The procedure worked! Go home and get a good night's rest." But by the time the couple arrived home, the phone was ringing again. "Come back *now!*" the nurse exclaimed.

Mark and Karen arrived at the hospital just minutes after Laura had died. When they walked in, Laura's eyes were open and her hand was outstretched. *You were waiting for me*, Mark thought. He held his daughter and said good-bye. How he longed to tell her how much he missed her and how he wanted to help her more than anything in the world.

"Laura, I'll think of you waiting for me just like on Father's Day—with your eyes wide open and your hands outstretched. Until that day, please know that there will always be a place in my heart where you and I will be holding hands."

Mark knew that he could not, on this earth, hold the hands of his first two children. Would he even have a chance to hold the hand of little Sarah? *Dear God*, he prayed, *how will I find the strength to endure this loss?*

The answer came. Holding hands with God was the only thing Mark could do. And so he did. Just as little Laura had reached out to him, Mark now reached out to God. He knew his grasp on God was tiny, but still he clung. He entrusted his remaining daughter's future into God's care.

Thirteen weeks later, Mark and Karen took Sarah home. They thanked God for their miracle as they sat on the sofa and held her. To their amazement, they soon discovered that Karen was pregnant again. A few days before Sarah's first birthday, God blessed them with Michael.

What an example of faith Mark and Karen are to me. Their journey through grief wasn't an easy one. Hiding, suffering, questioning, forgiving, and relating were all roadways of pain they walked. But seeking God through pain and suffering was their consistent response. Maybe that's what helped them move on and trust Him with the uncertainty of their future. Their actions have encouraged me to do the same—to reach out to God, place my uncertainty in His hands, and press on in my journey toward the future.

Are you willing to press on in your journey toward the future, or is it more comfortable to hide in a hole of despair?

Does fear have a grip on you? Does the thought of losing another child hold you captive to the past? *It's too painful to try again! I'm afraid I'll lose another child,* you think.

I understand some of what you are feeling. After every loss, I suffered deeply. That's why I allowed myself to journey through my grief at my own pace. So if you're not ready to face the future, that's okay. Seeking the future is just another part of the journey. It's up to you when you think you're ready to move on.

Is there hope after loss? Can faith overcome fear? Does God want you to trust Him and move on? Yes! But don't expect to feel as if you're "over your loss."

Be gentle with yourself. There will always be a part of your heart that holds hands with the child you never fully knew. You may still experience times when you cry, feel angry, or want to hide. That's okay. You lost a child, remember? But your loss has enlarged your life. Maybe you're more compassionate or less serious. Or perhaps you look at children as a gift now and don't take them for granted.

One thing is certain: you're not the same person you were. You've grown. Maybe it's time to grow some more. Are you ready to hold hands with the future? Look up.

God's eyes are open, and they're looking at *you.* He's watched you fight and struggle through your pain. He has been there the entire time and wants you to trust Him. He understands the anguish of your loss. He lost His Son too, remember? But His plan was that His loss would be our gain. He sent Jesus so that we could have eternal life.

Look up. His hand is outstretched. It's reaching for *you*. Please take it. Hold hands with Him, and trust Him with your future. He *is* your future. There is nothing too big for Him. With Him all things are possible.

God, facing the future is hard for me. I'm afraid I might lose another child. I feel as if my past is holding me captive. My uncertainty and doubts enslave me. If I try again, will I fail? What if I can never have another child? Is a child really Your will for me? Only You know what my future holds. Help me release my fear to You and replace it with faith. Even though I don't know what the future holds, I know who holds the future—You. Give me courage, Lord, as I take Your hand. Grasp it tightly, and never let go. I want to spend eternity with You and walk toward it, starting today. You are my future. It feels good to hold hands with You. With You I know I can face anything. Amen.

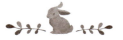

Steps Toward Healing

1. Is your past holding you captive from the future? If
   so, how?

   _____

   _____

   _____

   _____

   _____

2. God wants to strengthen you and help you. In what
   ways can you allow Him to hold your hand? In what
   ways can you allow others to hold your hand?

   _____

   _____

   _____

   _____

   _____

Devotion 29

JOURNEY THROUGH
THE GALLERY OF PRAISE

"See, I will create
new heavens and a new earth.
The former things will not be remembered,
nor will they come to mind.
But be glad and rejoice forever
in what I will create."

ISAIAH 65:17–18

*P*aintings adorn the walls of the museum. Each one is unique and tells a different story. Blue-green waves crash against the shore. Pastels and earth tones surround the cabin in the woods. Neon hues splash across the island sky. Golden flowers bloom on a cactus in the sand. Fluorescent zigzags of lightning illuminate the blackened sky behind a cross. White and yellow rays shine from the doorway of a tomb.

Can you hear the roar of the ocean? Can you feel the anger in the bolts behind the cross? Do you sense the peace and healing in the forest? Do you see hope beyond the empty tomb? You may feel as if your grief journey has led you to a gallery. Are the walls of your life adorned with emotional paintings of your grief that you've collected along the way?

Maybe you have one you've entitled *Anger*. The canvas shows a raging hurricane. You painted it right after you lost your child. Is there another one you call *Forgiving*? It shows a meadow with a rainbow in the sky. Your paintings may look different from mine, brushed with colors, experiences, relationships, and places I've never encountered.

One of the paintings from my life's gallery was completed the day before Mother's Day. It shows three pine trees and a stump. Mother's Day can be a happy-sad day for me. Although I had one living child at that time, I also had four children in heaven.

So when the men arrived to trim our trees, it never occurred to me that God was in the process of completing a painting in my life. One of our thirty-foot pine trees had grown too close to the fence and was becoming bothersome to our neighbor. We decided to have it cut down. This was a poignant decision for me because I love trees. As the men climbed to the top branches of the pine tree, it suddenly dawned on me that this living tree would soon be destroyed.

The buzz of chainsaws filled the air, and branches thumped to the ground. Sorrow breezed through my soul. The death of this tree was triggering my personal sense of loss. I began to weep. "Stop!" I cried out to the men. "Don't cut down the entire tree!" The men looked surprised. "Please leave a stump!" I sniffled. I wanted something visible to show for my loss.

With tears streaming down my face, I stared at my stump and prayed silently, *Lord, You are the Author of death and life. You are the Landscaper of my soul. I will give thanks and praise You in all circumstances!*

I knew this was a healing moment for me. I realized that the pathway to choose, in the midst of my pain that Mother's Day weekend, was the path of praising. I felt as if I had new eyes and could see beyond the pain to the Person who was with me through the pain.

Then I noticed that my stump was not alone. Three pine trees stood beside it. *How ironic!* I thought. *I've lost four children!* God had given me a loving reminder that He cares for me and understands the pain of my loss. He offered me a personal painting of three pine trees and a stump.

God calls you to examine each of the paintings of your grief and to find Him in each one. Is He your Comforter, Peace, Strength, Light, or Hope? Is He the Eye of the storm in the midst of your hurricane of anger or the God who keeps His rainbow of promises when you experience rainy days of grief? Go ahead! Look at your life's paintings. Now look beyond the paintings to who God is. Tell Him who He is to you. Repaint with new eyes; then journey through the gallery of praise.

God, my life is filled with emotional paintings I've collected along my grief journey. When I look at them, I recall my hurt and my pain. Give me new eyes. Help me see beyond each painting to who You are. I want to focus on You, not on my loss. You are the Creator of life and death. In my darkness, You are Light. In my fear, You are faithful. When I am confused, You are the way. You are my hope and future. Help me seek You and journey through my gallery with praise. Amen.

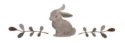

Steps Toward Healing

1. The gallery of your life is filled with emotional paintings. Share about your painting for each stage your journey—Hiding, Suffering, Questioning, and so on.

   _____

   _____

   _____

   _____

   _____

   _____

   _____

2. Now examine each painting. Do you see God there? Reflect on His strength in each of those areas. Praise Him for who He is. Perhaps a few new brushstrokes are in order.

   _____

   _____

   _____

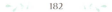

Devotion 30

SEEKING OTHERS BEFORE YOU, BESIDE YOU, BEHIND YOU

You then, my son, be strong in the grace
that is in Christ Jesus. And the things you
have heard me say in the presence of many
witnesses entrust to reliable people who
will also be qualified to teach others.

2 TIMOTHY 2:1–2

Where am I going and how do I get there? wondered Traveler as she stared at the desolate road that seemed to slither endlessly through the dark, barren valley. Instinctively she knew she must travel this route, though she yearned for another. Accompanied by Loneliness and Uncertainty, Traveler hesitated, then stepped onto the road. Her mood reflected the thundering sky as she trudged forward.

Several miles into her journey, the sky was nearly black. "I'm so weary; I can't go on!" she moaned as she rounded the bend. To her amazement, she saw a moving figure in the distance. She squeezed Uncertainty's hand as she hastened her steps and squinted at the enlarging figure.

"Hello! Who are you? Can you help me in my journey?" she shouted.

To her surprise, the figure stopped. Traveler edged closer and sensed that something significant was about to happen. The figure turned and thrust a weathered, calloused hand into Traveler's. The person's grip was firm and confident, as if to communicate, "I've been on this road a while, and I know where I'm going."

"I'm Mentor."

"Nice to meet you, Mentor. I'm Traveler. Have you been on this journey long?"

Mentor nodded as she wiped the perspiration from her brow. "I'm familiar with this road," she said as she gazed deep into Traveler's eyes. "Looks like you could use some company. Do you want to walk with me for a while?"

Traveler sighed. A sense of calm flooded her soul as she paced her stride with Mentor's.

She felt free to laugh, to cry, to share, and to probe for answers to her questions. Mile after mile, the duo trekked on. With each step, Traveler felt more confident. Hearing about the battles won, the lessons learned, and the mistakes made in Mentor's journey was like healing balm on the wounds of her heart. When Traveler stumbled and fell, Mentor quickly helped her up again. "You can make it!" Mentor cheered. With renewed hope, Traveler got back up and forged ahead, making sure to follow in Mentor's footsteps.

Night descended on the twosome, and fear taunted Traveler. "Hold on. Don't let go! I'll lead you!" Mentor exclaimed. Though weary, Traveler persevered and pressed on behind Mentor through the darkness to the sunrise.

The morning rays of sunshine revealed Others walking beside Traveler. *Where did they come from?* she wondered. Normally Traveler would have ignored them, but something within her urged her to start a conversation. She was amazed to discover that she and Others had much in common. Traveler hastened her pace and was surprised at the confidence she felt. *Maybe I'm stronger because I'm not alone in my journey,* she thought. *I have someone in front of me to guide me and others beside me to relate to and encourage me.*

What more could I need? wondered Traveler.

As if on cue in response to her thought, a scream pierced the air. "Hello! I'm lost and I don't know where I'm going. Will you help me?" Immediately Traveler stopped, turned, and looked at the path behind her. She knew what she must do.

Maybe you thought your grief journey would be over when you finished this book. I wish that were true. It may get easier, and at times you may not even think about your loss and be the person leading and walking beside others. But don't be surprised when you experience an unexpected outburst and find yourself retracing your steps and crying out for help.

Your road of grief is personal. It is a continuous journey. The scenery may change through the years and you may become wiser, but be gentle with yourself and give yourself permission to both give and receive support and guidance. God often teaches us more lessons just when we think we've learned everything we possibly could about our loss. His desire is that you press on toward eternity with truth in your heart and hope in your step.

Maybe it's time to ask God to use your loss for good. He knows exactly where you are in your journey and will provide the right people to help you grow. Look around.

God will show you who they are and will give you the courage and wisdom to reach out. Go ahead. You can do it!

God, thank You for providing others before me, beside me, and behind me in my grief journey to teach me and to help me grow. You understand how lonely the trek can be and how much I need to give and receive encouragement. Use my loss for good. In Your timing, help me take the hand of someone who has lost a child and needs hope. Be my mentor and companion as You work through me. Help me seek You and follow Your every step. Amen.

Steps Toward Healing

1. How can someone *before* you in grief guide you in your journey? Whose grief experience could you glean from? Share at least one way she could help you.

_____

_____

_____

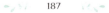

_____

_____

_____

2. Who are the people *beside* you? How do they
   support you?

_____

_____

_____

_____

_____

_____

3. Look back. Look around. Who is a few steps *behind*
   you in her journey through grief and needs your
   support? How will you reach out and help her?

_____

_____

_____

_____

_____

_____

Devotion 31

I'll Know My Child in Heaven

And I heard a loud voice from the throne saying, "Look! God's dwelling place is now among the people, and he will dwell with them. They will be his people, and God himself will be with them and be their God. 'He will wipe every tear from their eyes. There will be no more death' or mourning or crying or pain, for the old order of things has passed away."

REVELATION 21:3–4

I'm looking forward to heaven. No more corruption or death. No more tears or grieving. Unconditional love, truth, and wholeness will be the lifestyle. I'll be walking down streets of gold with a new body, heart, and mind. Crystal water from the river of life will flow down the middle of the street. And the Bible says there will even be trees!

Light will replace darkness. God Himself will illuminate heaven. I will experience perfect people in perfect fellowship. I can't even imagine what that will feel like. What fun it will be to reunite with friends and family who trusted Christ.

I wonder if Jesus will call me by name and welcome me personally into Paradise. With open arms and a loving smile, I can almost hear Him say, "Welcome home, Kathe!"

I hope that four green-eyed, grinning boys holding balloons will be standing next to Him—the children I never knew, the children I grieved. "Hi, Mom!" they'll shout. We'll hug and kiss, and then they'll take me by the hand and give me the heavenly tour. They'll introduce me to the angels, Moses, Hannah, the disciples, and Paul. We'll stop and have a picnic under the Tree of Life.

Then they'll guide me through a grove of pine trees to a brand-new mansion. How good it will feel to walk up the steps and realize I'm home at last and I never have to leave. And when I look at the children I never knew fully on earth, I'll realize this time there will be no good-byes, but eternity of praising God and getting to know them.

Heaven is a motivator to keep me pressing on in my journey through grief. Sometimes, like Paul in Philippians 1:23, my soul is homesick for my eternal home. Sometimes I long for those who have gone on ahead of me. Have you ever felt that way? What do you most look forward to in heaven? I bet you look forward to seeing Jesus. Do you hope your child is standing next to Him, waiting to greet you?

You'll finally understand fully why God allowed your child to enter eternity before you. Your whole perspective on life, death, and time will be made new. Your hiding, suffering, questioning, and need to forgive will vanish. The power of God's presence will overwhelm you. Your mourning will be replaced with dancing and eternal joy. You and I and the children we never knew will praise God for all of eternity.

Let's press on together in the journey to eternity and reach out to others who need the hope of heaven we have!

God, thank You for creating heaven. I can hardly wait to reach the end of my journey and hear You say, "Welcome home!" Thank You for creating an eternal place to live with no death or tears for those who know You personally. I'm assured of spending eternity with You in heaven because I believe that I am a sinner and that Jesus died on the cross for my sins, was buried, and rose again. How awesome it will be to finally thank Jesus face-to-face for what He did for me. I hope my child will be waiting with Him to greet me. Thank You for allowing me all of eternity to get to know the child You've always known. Help me press on in my earthly journey and seek You first in everything I do. Use me to shine the hope of heaven to others. Amen.

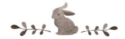

Steps Toward Healing

1. What do you most look forward to about heaven?

_____

_____

_____

_____

_____

2. What questions will you finally have answers to?

_____

_____

_____

_____

_____

3. How has your perspective on the loss of your child been changed by God during your journey?

_____

_____

_____

_____

_____

Read more about heaven: Isaiah 35:10; 65:17; Ezekiel 1:26–28; Luke 15:10; John 3:5–7; 14:2–3; 1 Corinthians 15:36–38; Philippians 3:20–21; 1 Thessalonians 4:16–17; 2 Timothy 4:8; Hebrews 12:22–23; Revelation 15:2–3; 20:1–22:5.

Part 7

SHARING YOUR STORY

But in your hearts revere Christ as Lord. Always
be prepared to give an answer to everyone who
asks you to give the reason for the hope that you
have. But do this with gentleness and respect.

1 PETER 3:15

Sharing your story can be a healing part of your journey. You may be thinking, *But it's too painful*, or, *Who would want to hear my story?* I'm amazed by the people I encounter at the grocery store, in our neighborhood, on an airplane, or through a friend of a friend who also lost a child and need personal encouragement. God knows exactly who I need to meet. He may choose a small group setting for you to share your story, or He may choose for you to share with a large auditorium of people. What's important is having a willing heart to trust and obey Him when He calls you to share with someone.

Even though I frequently share with others, each time I share the story of my loss, my stomach churns and the scar of my heart rips open again. That's normal for me and keeps me relying on God's power. I have discovered that it is during those weak times that God does His best work. When I am weak, He is strong—and God's Holy Spirit empowers me to do or say things I thought were impossible (2 Corinthians 12:7–10; Ephesians 3:20).

One day a woman stopped me in the parking lot and asked, "Oh, I see you had your baby!" I could tell she had no idea I had lost our child. This was an opportunity to share my personal journey and share about God's sustaining power. Did anything spectacular occur? Not really, at least from my human viewpoint. But later, when I saw her in the store, she knew my name and we always talked. When she experienced difficulty, she sought me out. When she had questions about God, yep, you guessed it—she asked me. My husband and I have numerous stories of our "grief encounters" with others. God wants to work through me and use my story of losing a child to touch others and point them to Him. And He wants to do the same through you. What an awesome privilege we have. For me, it gives eternal purpose to my pain and validates the life of the children I never knew.

So get ready! When someone opens the door of conversation to talk about loss . . . share your story! The purpose in doing so is to give others hope in specific ways through your grief experience. When you share how God has worked in your life through your loss, you will encourage others.

How can you best prepare to share? My friend Carol Kent helped me tell my story verbally and in written form through her annual Speak Up Conference and her book *Speak Up with Confidence: A Step-by-Step Guide for Speakers* (NavPress). Both tools give a practical how-to approach to communicating your story. I've adapted her guidelines to help you begin writing your grief story. I've discovered that writing down my life lessons prepares me to speak them. It's your turn . . . You can do it!

1. Start with prayer. Ask for God's wisdom and discernment in what to share.
2. Identify one personal experience in your journey through grief when God has worked through your life.
3. Briefly share what happened. Were you hiding, suffering, questioning, forgiving, relating, seeking?

4. What emotions did you experience? Did you feel angry, confused, sad, guilty, lonely, depressed, hopeless?

5. What spiritual lesson did you learn from it? If you were holding a grudge against your doctor, did God show the importance of forgiveness?

6. What Scripture verses or passages apply?

7. How can your story encourage others in a specific way? Revisit your gallery of praise (Devotion 29). Is there a painting hanging on the wall that could lead someone to praise God? Picture how God might use you. Here is one example of picturing the end result: "I want to help those who have lost a child understand the need to forgive others who have hurt them and the benefits of forgiving so that they will identify at least one person this week and practice forgiveness."

❧ A PRAYER GUIDE ❧
FOR SPECIAL DAYS

*P*rayer is a powerful gift you can give or receive. Allow God's Word to be your (or others') prayer guide on days or occasions when you need encouragement. Choose from the variety of topics and scriptures adapted to be your poignant personalized prayer.

When You Face Mother's Day or Father's Day

The Lord bless _____
and keep _____ ;
The Lord make His face shine on _____
and be gracious to _____ ;
The Lord turn His face toward _____
and give _____ *peace.*

FROM NUMBERS 6:24–26

When You Face Your Due Date

God, You are _____'s hiding place; protect _____ from trouble and surround _____ with songs of deliverance.

FROM PSALM 32:7

When You Face a Medical Procedure

God, cover _____ with Your feathers, and under Your wings help _____ to find refuge; may Your faithfulness be _____'s shield and rampart.

FROM PSALM 91:4

When You Face a Baby Shower/ Baptism/Dedication

Create in _____ a pure heart, O God, and renew a steadfast spirit within _____. Do not cast _____ from Your presence or take Your Holy Spirit from _____. Restore to _____ the joy of Your salvation and grant _____ a willing spirit, to sustain _____.

FROM PSALM 51:10–12

When Someone You Know
Becomes Pregnant or Has a Baby

*Lord, protect _____ from envy
and selfish ambition. Give _____
wisdom from heaven that is pure, peace-loving,
considerate, submissive, full of mercy and good
fruit, impartial and sincere.*

FROM JAMES 3:16–17

When You Face Holidays/
Family Gatherings

*Clothe _____ with compassion,
kindness, humility, gentleness, and patience.
Help _____ bear
with others and forgive whatever grievances
_____ may have against others. Help
_____ forgive as You, Lord, forgave. Help
_____ put on love, which binds them all
together in perfect unity. Let the peace of Christ
rule in _____'s heart, since as members
of one body _____ is called to peace.*

FROM COLOSSIANS 3:12–15

When You Are Ovulating

Your love, Lord, reaches to the heavens, Your faithfulness to the skies. Your righteousness is like the highest mountains, Your justice like the great deep. You, Lord, preserve both people and animals. How priceless is Your unfailing love, O God! Help _____ take refuge in the shadow of Your wings.

FROM PSALM 36:5–7

When You and Your Spouse Disagree

Help _____ bear with _____ and forgive whatever grievances _____ may have against _____. Help _____ do, whether in word or deed, all in the name of the Lord Jesus, giving thanks to God the Father through Him.

FROM COLOSSIANS 3:13, 17

I pray that _____ will speak the truth in love to _____.

FROM EPHESIANS 4:15

When You Start Your Period

Lord, Your Word says that You go before _____ *and You will be with* _____*; You will never leave* _____ *or forsake* _____. *Help* _____ *not be afraid or discouraged.*

FROM DEUTERONOMY 31:8

When You Have Questions About Having Another Child

God, You know the plans You have for _____, *plans to prosper* _____ *and not to harm* _____, *plans to give* _____ *hope and a future. Help* _____ *call on You and pray to You, and You will listen to* _____. *I pray* _____ *will seek You and find You when* _____ *seeks You with all* _____*'s heart.*

FROM JEREMIAH 29:11–13

When Your Pregnancy Test Is Negative

God, help _____ lift up _____'s eyes and look to the heavens and know who created all these. You bring out the starry host one by one, and call forth each of them by name. Because of Your great power and mighty strength, not one of them is missing. Help _____ know that You are the everlasting God, the Creator of the ends of the earth. You will not grow weary and you will give _____ strength.

FROM ISAIAH 40:26–29

When Your Pregnancy Test Is Positive

Help _____ be strong and courageous. Do not allow _____ to be afraid or discouraged, for You, Lord, will be with _____ and _____'s unborn child wherever _____ goes.

FROM JOSHUA 1:9

*Let _____ fix _____'s
eyes on Jesus, the pioneer and perfecter of faith.*

FROM HEBREWS 12:2

When You Feel Alone or Misunderstood

*Help _____ trust You with all of _____'s
heart and lean not on _____'s own
understanding. In all of _____'s ways may
_____ acknowledge You, Lord, and
You will direct _____'s steps.*

FROM PROVERBS 3:5–6

*You, Lord, go before _____. You, the
God of Israel, be _____'s rear guard.*

FROM ISAIAH 52:12

*Show _____ Your ways, Lord, teach
_____ Your paths. Guide _____
in Your truth and teach _____, for
You are _____'s God and Savior, and
_____'s hope is in You all day long.*

FROM PSALM 25:4–5

When You Face the Anniversary of Your Child's Birth/Death

Let _____ wait patiently for You, Lord; turn to _____ and hear _____'s cry. Lift _____ out of the slimy pit, out of the mud and mire. Set _____'s feet on a rock and give _____ a firm place to stand. Put a new song in _____'s mouth.

FROM PSALM 40:1–3

Strengthen _____ and help _____. Uphold _____ with Your righteous right hand.

FROM ISAIAH 41:10

When Your Doctor Disappoints You

See to it that no one takes _____ captive through hollow and deceptive philosophy, which depends on human tradition and the elemental spiritual forces of this world rather than on Christ.

FROM COLOSSIANS 2:8

Help _____ say like Jesus did, "Father, forgive them, for they do not know what they are doing."

FROM LUKE 23:34

When You Are Weary from Waiting

Help _____ know _____'s times are in Your hands.

FROM PSALM 31:15

Help _____ glory in _____'s sufferings because we know that suffering produces perseverance; perseverance, character; and character, hope.

FROM ROMANS 5:3–4

Help _____ hope for what _____ does not yet have and wait patiently.

FROM ROMANS 8:25

This is the day that the Lord has made; let _____ rejoice and be glad in it.

FROM PSALM 118:24

✦ Discussion Guide ✦

The following eight sessions correspond with sections in the book and may be used in a variety of settings and time frames to meet your needs. Each session contains four questions and an assignment for the next week's session. You may also add additional questions from the "Steps Toward Healing" questions at the end of each devotion.

You may choose to use this as a six- to eight-week series, for a weekend retreat, or in a more intimate setting with another person or a small group to dig deeper. Because grief is personal and can't be confined to a method or timeframe, it's important to use this only as a guide; be flexible and adjust as God guides you. Pray and ask Him to help you in your journey.

Session 1: Introduction

1. Introduce yourself. Who are you, and why are you here?
2. Read the Introduction on pages xvii–xxii.
3. In the roller coaster analogy, which group of riders can you most identify with? Enthusiastic? Cautious? In between? Sick? Why?

4. The author's prayer is that her book (and this discussion) will point you to God and help you experience His presence in the midst of your pain. How have you already experienced God in midst of your pain? What do you hope you receive from this group? (Write every group member's comment down, and make this a closing prayer for this session.)

5. Homework: Read Part 1: Hiding.

Session 2: Hiding

1. How did you experience God in the midst of your pain since we last met?

2. What story, verse, example, or questions in the section on hiding spoke to your heart? Why?

3. Hiding started in the garden of Eden. Read Genesis 3:8–9. Personalize these verses by inserting your name. How have you or others been hiding from your loss?

4. Psalm 43:3 says, "Send out your light and your truth; let them guide me" (NLT). What steps can you take this week to be truthful to yourself and with others?

5. Homework: Read Part 2: Suffering.

Session 3: Suffering

1. How did you experience God in the midst of your pain since we last met?
2. What story, verse, example, or questions in the section on suffering spoke to your heart? Why?
3. Read Romans 5:3–5. What does this verse say that suffering produces?
4. How do the examples of David, Hannah, and Jesus encourage you in your suffering?
5. Homework: Read Part 3: Questioning.

Session 4: Questioning

1. How did you experience God in the midst of your pain since we last met?
2. What story, verse, example, or questions in the section on questioning spoke to your heart? Why?
3. In devotion 11, the author says that "what we believe about God during those times of uncertainty will influence how we respond. If we believe that our circumstance is something Satan slipped by God when He wasn't looking, we will plummet to the depths and drown in despair. But if we view the God of the Bible as sovereign, supreme, and the One who calms the waters, we will be buoyed with hope. We will see purpose, even

though we may not know now what the purpose is." What questions do you still have that remain unanswered about your loss? Who has answers?

4. God said in Hebrews 13:5, "Never will I leave you; never will I forsake you." How does the promise of His presence comfort you in your uncertainty?

5. Homework: Read Part 4: Forgiving.

Session 5: Forgiving

1. How did you experience God in the midst of your pain since we last met?

2. What story, verse, example, or questions in the section on forgiving spoke to your heart? Why?

3. Is there someone who has hurt you that you need to confront and offer forgiveness to? Is there someone you have hurt and you need to seek forgiveness? How will you take steps to do this?

4. Are you angry with God about your loss and feel as if He should have intervened? Forgiving God doesn't mean He's guilty because He can't commit sin. Sometimes our false expectations get in the way of what we think God should have done to prevent our loss. How have yours?

5. Homework: Read Part 5: Relating.

Session 6: Relating

1. How did you experience God in the midst of your pain since we last met?

2. What story, verse, example, or questions in the section on relating spoke to your heart? Why?

3. Who has God brought into your life that can relate to your loss? How does this make you feel?

4. Second Corinthians 1:3–4 says we are to comfort others with the comfort we have received. How have you received comfort from others, and how can you give it?

5. Homework: Read Part 6: Seeking.

Session 7: Seeking

1. How did you experience God in the midst of your pain since we last met?

2. What story, verse, example, or questions in the section on seeking spoke to your heart? Why?

3. God may have special work for you to do in spite of your loss. Which of the examples of the contemporary women from Devotion 27 encouraged you? How could God use your loss for good? What ideas do you have?

4. Heaven is a real place where your child lives. How can you be assured you will go to heaven and see your child again? John 3:16 says, "For God so loved the

world that he gave his one and only Son, that whoever believes in him shall not perish but have eternal life."

5. Homework: Read Part 7: Sharing Your Story.

Session 8: Sharing Your Story

1. Review your hoped-for outcome of this group from session 1. What did you desire? Did you receive what you hoped for from this group?

2. How did you experience God through your pain?

3. Share one personal experience in your journey through grief where God has worked through your life.

4. What spiritual lesson did you learn from it?

5. What do you sense God is asking you to do next?

SCRIPTURE INDEX

Genesis 3:8–9 . . . . 2, 209

Numbers 6:24–26 119

Deuteronomy 31:8 203

Joshua 1:9 . . . . 77, 204

Ruth 1:20–21 105

1 Samuel 1:8 51

1 Kings 3:16–28 16

2 Chronicles 20:6 75

Job 28:20, 23 30

Psalm 1:3 137

Psalm 4 81

Psalm 5 27

Psalm 16 87

Psalm 17 87

Psalm 22:19 35

Psalm 23 87

Psalm 25:4–5 205

Psalm 31:15 207

Psalm 32:7 . . . . 6, 200

Psalm 32:8 10

Psalm 36:5–7 202

Psalm 38:4 72

Psalm 40:1–3 . . . . 80, 206

Psalm 43:3 . . . . 11, 209

Psalm 44:20–21 40

Psalm 46 27

Psalm 46:10 23

Psalm 51:10–12 200

Psalm 91:4 200

Psalm 118:24 207

Psalm 139 22

Psalm 139:1, 15 18

Psalm 139:15–16 1

Psalm 139:23–24 90

Psalm 142:7 103

Psalm 147:3 164

Proverbs 3:5–6 205

Ecclesiastes 11:5 59

Isaiah 35:10 193

Isaiah 40:26–29 204

Isaiah 41:10 . . . . 94, 170, 206

Isaiah 43:2 60

Isaiah 46:9–10 75

Isaiah 52:12 205

Isaiah 65:17 193

Isaiah 65:17–18 178

Jeremiah 29:11–13 203

Jeremiah 29:11–14 158

Ezekiel 1:26–28 193

Malachi 3:6 46

Matthew 5:4 51
Matthew 7:7 157
Matthew 10:29–30 75
Matthew 10:29–31 131
Matthew 11:28 27
Matthew 11:28–29 81
Matthew 16:13, 16 126
Mark 2:7. 109
Luke 6:20–49 81
Luke 15:10. 193
Luke 23:34 . . . . 92, 95, 207
John 3:5–7 193
John 3:16 . . . . 116, 119, 212
John 5 168
John 5:6 165
John 5:8–9 105
John 11 82
John 11:4 79
John 11:21. 79
John 13:34. 144
Romans 3:23 119
Romans 5:3–4 207
Romans 5:3–5 210
Romans 8:25 207
Romans 15:13. 149
1 Corinthians 15:36–38 193
2 Corinthians 1:3–4 125
2 Corinthians 10:5 112

2 Corinthians 12:7–10 196
Galatians 6:2 147
Ephesians 3:20 196
Ephesians 4:15 202
Ephesians 4:31 65
Ephesians 4:32 147
Philippians 1:6 218
Philippians 1:23 191
Philippians 3:20–21 193
Philippians 4:13 94
Colossians 2:8 206
Colossians 3:12–15. 201
Colossians 3:13 88
Colossians 3:13, 17. 202
1 Thessalonians 4:16–17. 193
1 Thessalonians 4:18. 147
2 Timothy 2:1–2 183
2 Timothy 4:8. 193
Hebrews 12:2 205
Hebrews 12:22–23 193
Hebrews 13:5 . . . . 80, 211
James 3:16–17. 201
1 Peter 3:15 144
1 Peter 5:7. 25
1 John 1:9 108
Revelation 15:2–3 193
Revelation 20:1–22:5. 193
Revelation 21:3–4 189

A NOTE FROM THE AUTHOR

*A*re you over it yet?"

Those words still make me cringe, even though many years have passed now. I will never get over losing my children, though I wish it were that simple. My wounded heart is *healing*, but it still has a scar.

Will the scar from my losses ever fully heal? Maybe not in this lifetime, but in heaven it will. It's hard to believe this book was first released in 2001. I am humbled by the thousands of readers around the world who have journeyed through its pages. I've wiped away a few happy-sad tears as I've stepped back through the pages of my life. For now, God has opened my heart to a new understanding of who He is through the people, stories, places, and circumstances He allowed me to encounter. He is my Hopelifter, my Healer, and my life's Editor.

Thank you for taking the time to journey with me. As you continue to step forward to grieve the child you never knew, I pray you will have renewed perspective and hope. Your child matters and will continue to have an impact in the world. Take a moment to write your child's name on the dedication page at the front of the book.

I am grateful to those past and present who encouraged me in writing or updating this book. I am humbled by the multitudes of readers and leaders worldwide who validated the need for this book and have given it as a gift of comfort or used it to lead a grief support group since its original release in 2001.

A special thanks to:

My prayer team; my mom; my fellow ministry leaders who have lost children and have gathered around my dining room table to share your hearts, tears, prayers, and resources to reach out together to help grieving moms; my friends in the fire; my doctor; my friends, supporters and mentors for reasons or seasons; my fellow grieving moms on my bus trips; my 2001 Zondervan family and my 2015 HarperCollins family; my sons, Jake, Josh, and Jordan, who gave me hope; my husband, Rich, who willingly started many days in tears by reading every devotion.

And to you, the reader: thank you for opening the pages of this book. When I felt discouraged and wanted to give up, I kept picturing you reading this book, seeking comfort for your soul. Behind every name or story is another story. And behind the names and stories is a personal God who

Samuel Sable Maddie Maxie Baby

Seth Jericho Sam James Peter Baby

Alyssa Kiara Gracie Lily Ember Holl

Morgan Laura Linda Rachel Kristi

Kelsey Joshua Tina Scott Jodi Garr

Molly Baby Young Baby Miller Ba

Baby Perry Reed Daniel Baby Sank

Baby Emmorey Baby Gritter Baby

Baby Kent Baby Bullock Baby F

Austin Rebekah Gregory Baby Moo

Lisa Evan Holly Gary Katelyn Baby

Baby Nichols Baby Carpenter Baby